Foundations of Yoga

"In *Foundations of Yoga*, Basile P. Catoméris presents a comprehensive view of the ancient practice of Yoga through the eyes of a present-day yogi. Those interested in the roots of yogic philosophy and practice will find his clear explanations informative and enlightening."

BIFF MITHOEFER, INTERNATIONAL YOGA TEACHER AND AUTHOR OF *THE YIN YOGA KIT* AND COAUTHOR OF *THE THERAPEUTIC YOGA KIT*

"It is with the greatest pleasure that I recommend Basile P. Catoméris's book *Foundations of Yoga*. Sri Shyam Sundar Goswami and his understanding and practical application of Hatha Yoga has been instrumental in spreading this form of Yoga in the West. The increased interest in the practice of Hatha Yoga in Europe and the United States makes this book especially important."

OLLE QVARNSTRÖM, PROFESSOR OF INDIC RELIGIONS, LUND UNIVERSITY, SWEDEN

Foundations of Yoga

The Traditional Teachings of Sri Shyam Sundar Goswami

BASILE P. CATOMÉRIS

Inner Traditions
Rochester, Vermont • Toronto, Canada

Inner Traditions
One Park Street
Rochester, Vermont 05767
www.InnerTraditions.com

SUSTAINABLE FORESTRY INITIATIVE Certified Sourcing www.sfiprogram.org SFI-00854

Text Stock is SFI certified

Library of Congress Cataloging-in-Publication Data

Catoméris, Basile P.

Foundations of yoga : the traditional teachings of Sri Shyam Sundar Goswami / Basile P. Catoméris.

pages ; cm

Includes index.

ISBN 978-1-59477-454-6 (pbk.) — ISBN 978-1-59477-511-6 (e-book)

1. Goswami, Shyam Sundar. 2. Hatha yoga. 3. Yoga—Philosophy. 4. Hindu philosophy. I. Title.

RA781.7.C39 2013

613.7'046—dc23

2012017324

Printed and bound in the United States by Lake Book Manufacturing, Inc.
The text stock is SFI certified. The Sustainable Forestry Initiative® program promotes sustainable forest management.

10 9 8 7 6 5 4 3 2 1

Text design and layout by Virginia Scott Bowman
This book was typeset in Garamond Premier Pro with Bodoni Antigua and Gill Sans used as display typefaces

For more information about Shyam Sundar Goswami and the Goswami Yoga Institute, please visit the institute's website at **www.goswamiyogainstitute.com**.

Contents

Foreword

Gunnar Adler-Karlsson

In his introduction to this book, Basile P. Catoméris mentions that Professor S. S. Goswami attracted thousands of pupils to his Yoga school in Stockholm. Fortunately, I was one of the lucky ones. At the beginning of the 1960s, I overexerted myself on an academic book concerning the extremely sensitive and secret economic side of the Cold War, became a bit nervous, and went to a doctor. The only fault he found was that I had worked too hard with my mind, neglecting my body. He gave me the address of the Goswami school.

Since then I have had close encounters with a number of statesmen and Nobel Prize winners. But I have never in my life met an individual with a stronger charisma combined with such a wonderful mixture of empathy, warm humor, and profound seriousness as Sri Shyam Sundar Goswami. His Haṭha Yoga exercises, together with some deep meditation, quickly picked up both my physical and mental state. For over forty years since then, few weeks have passed without my doing a serious Yoga exercise.

I have no doubt that it was Professor Goswami's Yoga teaching that gave me the strength to overcome those difficulties in life that all truth-seeking—that is, provocative—individuals are bound to meet. In this superstressed modern world I don't hesitate to advise anybody and everybody to devote a few hours a week to Haṭha Yoga. All the other hours will benefit from it, and you will enjoy a stronger body and a quicker, as well as more relaxed, mind.

Lest the reader think I am a fundamentalist Yoga fanatic, let me just mention that an English translation of the title of my latest book in Swedish could be "Memories of an Inflated Bacteria." This scientifically fully correct phrase is a reminder of Goswami's Indian wisdom, *tat twam asi*: "you are it"—you are the great-great-great grandchild of the first bacteria at the beginning of life on this wonderful planet.

My own memory of and gratitude to Sri Shyam Sundar Goswami will continue until the other bacteria seriously start to consume me.

Preface

Yoga is the inseparable heart of the Hindu school of thought. It is said, "There is no Yoga without Hinduism and no Hinduism without Yoga." On the other hand, the renowned father of analytical psychology, Carl G. Jung, described Yoga as "one of the greatest things the human mind has ever created."

Yoga is a vast subject. Moreover, a serious study of it cannot limit itself to a fragmentary account of its techniques and methods, as is too often the case today. The study of Yoga effectively requires a broad, and above all accurate, understanding of the different aspects of Yoga: spiritual, metaphysical, and philosophical, as well as its conception of human psychology. The original literature on Yoga consisted of manuscripts primarily written in Sanskrit, which were the fruit of interpretations by its practitioners, who were intuitive and empirical and, at the same time, faithful and enlightened.

These days, there is no rule or formal requirement for the teaching of Yoga. A liberal attitude of this kind, together with the popularization of this precious source of human knowledge, has resulted in the circulation of numerous misunderstandings about and amalgams of the nature, traditional values, and objectives of Yoga. Numerous self-proclaimed "masters," either because of naiveté or lack of respect for a sacred tradition, have failed to obtain serious theoretical and practical training; as a result they pass along ineptitudes and untruths.

Sometimes they claim an altruistic motivation; often they reveal overtly mercantile ambitions. It should be noted, moreover, that representatives of very honorable professions, in a learned manner supported by rational analysis, laud the benefits of such or such an *āsana* or posture, thus encouraging less aware individuals to take an à la carte approach to something that in fact constitutes a whole—a holistic doctrine that requires an integrated approach.

In the wake of the ongoing Yoga renaissance, a plethora of Yoga schools with various *āsana* management programs has emerged all over the world. On several worldwide traveling occasions, I had the opportunity to assess how *āsanas* are interpreted in various Yoga schools and ashrams of India, Europe, the United States, and the Middle East. Quite impartially, and with due respect to the managers of Yoga schools and institutions, whether they are promoting Hindu culture, business-oriented, or just dilettante, I must say that I found the most intelligent, methodically designed *āsana* training at the Goswami Yoga institute of Stockholm, Sweden, reportedly Europe's oldest Yoga school. There pupils can discover a complete use of traditional *āsanas* that have been rationally adapted to meet the needs of urban practitioners. Four different courses are available: an all-round program involving virtually the whole musculature, a program of essentially static *āsanas,* one course called Mahā Mudrā with an anaerobic training of the lungs, as well as an intensive program with emphasis on the heart and the lungs. This program embraces the complete range of human physical activity: flexibility, strength, speed, and endurance.

On another note, more formal but nevertheless representative of an offense consistent with the level of ignorance, indeed disdain, that is accorded to traditions, is the frequent abuse of the term *guru.* Sacred in India, the holy teachers who are addressed with this term are done a disservice by the indiscriminate use of the word in the West, where it is used to refer to the worst alongside the best, notably the leaders of sects that have little to recommend them or in some cases are even contemptible.

It is to dispel numerous such mistaken ideas that I am presenting to the English reader a synthesis of Yoga according to the oral and written teachings of Sri Shyam Sundar Goswami, an incontrovertible Yoga master, who is nevertheless unknown in many parts of the West. *Foundations of Yoga* is intended to express an "Indo-European's" indebtedness and to bear witness to my profound loyalty, which is inseparable from my immense debt of gratitude to one of India's great spiritual sons.

Here it is useful to specify the nature and role of the yogi as one who has, in the Hindu tradition, attained the state of *samādhi,** an epiphanic experience (in the etymological sense of the term) of a state of immediate insight that reveals the essence of a given object to the subject. A yogi (or yogini) is not necessarily a guru or a learned person, yet in India yogi(ni)s enjoy a high social status. It is said that wealthy and mighty maharajas of lore would search for the presence of a yogi(ni) in their genealogy to reinforce their noble lineage. There are numerous yogis in India who do not wish to appear in public or to reveal the fruit of their spiritual experiences, even to those close to them.

A yogi often lives with a minimum of comfort. In some cases, he leads an ascetic life, like that of an anchorite or hermit. He is able to endure deprivations of all kinds and to brave the elements, both extreme heat and the cold that is found in isolated areas of the Himalayas. Yogis and yoginis of this kind primarily devote themselves to an all-absorbing introspective research that excludes even the idea of comfort or any desire to become actively involved in the affairs of the surrounding world.

However, it is not accurate to conclude that a yogi is necessarily an asocial being, for a different example can be seen in the famous *naga naga* ascetics, whose tradition goes back three thousand years. This very special category of God seekers follows the pragmatic philosophy that is Yoga, which is to Hinduism what spirituality is to religion—it's ontological raison d'être. They form a spiritual elite composed of men and occasionally women; their bodies are kept naked, except for a thin layer of oil and sandalwood ashes, and these exceptional men are masters of self-defense. In former times, these ascetics, who are both venerated and

*A glossary of Sanskrit and other technical terms is provided for the reader's convenience at the end of the book.

feared, did not hesitate to come to the rescue of a nearby village that had been invaded by a hostile tribe.

But there are also yogis who practice a less rigorous asceticism and are fully integrated into the society in which they live. Some are content with a revealed or intellectual interpretation of the sacred writings that form the basis of Yoga. Others keep the oral tradition of Yoga alive, giving an account of their experiences, which they pass on with a unique flair. These yogis transmit this knowledge to whoever expresses a wish for it, according to the level and qualifications of the person. Yogic teaching is generally given without any discrimination of sex, caste, nationality, or religion.

For these spiritual heirs of an ancient tradition, the actions and attitudes implied by the word *proselytism,* in all its connotations, positive or negative, are unthinkable. Strengthened by a heritage that has overcome the vicissitudes of many civilizations, past and present, these yogis escape the grip of the usual ideological phenomena disseminated by monotheistic religions, which they refuse to imitate.

Foundations of Yoga exposes briefly the four paths of classical Yoga: Mantra Yoga, Hatha Yoga, Laya Yoga, and Raja Yoga. Specific paths that are also included in what is known as the "royal path" of Yoga—namely Jñāna Yoga, Bhakti Yoga, Karma Yoga, and Kriya Yoga—will only be alluded to. The current work is distinguished from most of the numerous books that have recently appeared with wellness as the main target, which not infrequently include alternative therapies whose advertised results too often have as yet to be evidenced. Focusing mainly on the philosophical background of traditional Yoga in India, this book does not provide practical directions for the practice of Yoga. Those who wish to be properly guided in the path of modern Yoga by an authentic Yoga master may read the latest edition of Sri S. S. Goswami's *Advanced Hatha Yoga* (Inner Traditions, 2012).

In keeping with the serious treatment of Yoga presented in this book, certain technical terms are used, which, in their English translation (sometimes employing neologisms), might at first glance seem strange and hermetic, solely because there is no equivalent in Western culture. The reader will hopefully not allow himself or herself to be put off by such terms, which, for example, offer technical descriptions of numerous states of consciousness that, in the yogi's view, open new horizons beyond the three known states of waking, sleeping, and dreaming.

It should be noted that, to avoid all misunderstanding, the author has preferred to use the expression *mental concentration,* instead of the vague terms *meditation* and *contemplation,* to designate the key method that results in the three states of *dhāraṇā, dhyāna,* and *samādhi.*

Moreover, the imprecision and indeed the ambiguity of the terms *thought, spirit, soul,* or *psyche* explains the adoption of the term *mind,* which will generally be used to designate the mental faculties, notably the intellect, the emotions, and the will. Finally, the meaning of the word *thought* will be limited to ideas, images, sensations, and other forms of nonphysical perception.

In the absence of unequivocal rules in the question of the transcription of Sanskrit, and in order to facilitate reading, the author has adopted a simplified style of transliteration, employing some diacritical marks, detailed in a pronunciation guide that appears at the conclusion of the text. In addition, proper nouns are written with capital letters, unlike Sanskrit, which does not make this distinction; other Sanskrit terms are shown in lowercase italics throughout. Finally, there is the use of plurals, a form that is not found in Sanskrit and that may be seen by pure philologists as an incongruity.

May Yoga practitioners temporarily release themselves of all judgment in reading this book, which has no other ambition than to set out an authentic teaching that is traditional and faithful to the universality of Yoga, a teaching that is purged of all belief and ideology.

May the reader appreciate the axiom according to which book knowledge, as advanced as it is, will never be able to answer the natural need of a human being to find inner peace and harmony, which constitutes the real goal of philosophy. May each also realize the truth of the wisest of precepts, which, in the ancient Delphic oracle, offered itself to the contemplation of every passerby: *Γνῶθι σεαυτόν,* "Know yourself." This piece of wisdom is also found in the Hindu teachings of the Kaṭha Upaniṣad: "Stand up, wake up, and, with the grace of a spiritual guide, learn who you are."

Acknowledgments

This work is dedicated to my spiritual parents, Sri Shyam Sundar Goswami and Ma Santi Devi Roy. I also wish to express my heartfelt gratitude to all the people and friends who in various ways contributed to the realization of this book.

A special thanks to the memory of late Jonathan Collins, for a fruitful collaboration in translating my original French text. Many thanks to Alain Rolland for his artwork on *āsanas* and Marc Rattray for his suggestions. My blessings go to faithful *cela* and friend Dr. Buddhadeb Chaudury, whose keen interest in my own dharmic work has been a most appreciated source of inspiration.

Heartiest thanks to most faithful disciples Guita Tiselius, Eva Olandersson, Renée Lord, and Abdullah Hassan. Their very presence and friendly support have inspired me all along in providing practitioners and teachers of Yoga a written, reliable account of the pragmatic philosophy of Haṭha Yoga. My sincere appreciation to Edit Edery for her willingness to illustrate most of the *āsanas* displayed in the book.

I also wish to express my sincere appreciation to acquisitions editor Jon Graham, who never lost confidence in the viability of this book project, and my deep gratitude for the excellent work of Inner Traditions' editors Nancy Yeilding and Laura Schlivek.

INTRODUCTION

At the Feet of the "Lion of Bengal"

The sole intention of the present treatise is to describe faithfully, without claiming to be exhaustive or perfect, an oral teaching in the initiatory tradition, in this case by an authentic Yoga master. Sri Shyam Sundar Goswami was exceptional in many ways, as much for his physical force as for his spirituality, accompanied by a remarkable faculty of exegesis. He devoted his life exclusively to the practice, study, research, and teaching of Yoga. In *The Deeper Dimension of Yoga* (Shambhala Publications, 2003). Dr. Georg Feuerstein, an author who is as prolific as he is eminent, quotes Sri Goswami among the personalities to whom the modern world owes its practice of Haṭha Yoga.

The Haṭha yogi Sachindra Kumar C. Majumdar, author of the book *Introduction to Yoga Principles and Practices* (Pelham Books Ltd., 1967), gives a brief history of modern Yoga with a rare objectivity when he writes:

> The scientific and creative interpretation of Haṭha Yoga in our time is due principally to the work of two distinguished yogis: Yogi Madhavdas and Shyam Sundar Goswami . . . [the latter] is deeply versed in both Western and Eastern methods of physical education. . . .

> [He] has written a book . . . entitled *Haṭha Yoga: an Advanced Method of Physical Education and Concentration.* This work is modern, cogent and the most comprehensive, definitive treatment of Yoga to be found in the Western world today. It is also the most completely illustrated book.

The Life of Sri Shyam Sundar Goswami

Born on October 11, 1891, in Santipur, West Bengal, India, an area where numerous philosophical and cultural celebrities saw the light of day, Shyam Sundar Goswami comes from an ancient lineage that goes back more than seven centuries. One of his ancestors was the guru (spiritual guide) of King Hatnabati and the successor of the famous *bhakti* yogi Caitanya. In India, the name Goswami is inseparable from the goal of scholarship and teaching.

Shyam Sundar Goswami was a weak child, predisposed to illness. As a result he tried, with little success, several systems of physical education, both Eastern and Western, that were supposed to enable him to reinforce his immune system. But only when he was guided and initiated into the discipline of Haṭha Yoga by Balaka Bharati, a hermit yogi with extraordinary powers, was the young Goswami able to improve his health, reinforce his immune system, and develop extraordinary power and control in both the physical and mental realms.

Shyam Sundar Goswami did not distinguish himself solely in the discipline of Haṭha Yoga. Following his meeting in Kolkata (formerly Calcutta) with Sri Dijwapada Sharma, a master of Laya Yoga, he also excelled in this other fundamental and reputedly challenging path of Yoga.* His qualities, to which one should add his erudition and brilliance, procured him the honorary title of "Lion of Bengal."

After teaching Haṭha Yoga in Kolkata, Shyam Sundar Goswami, accompanied by his disciple Dr. Dinabandhu Pramanick, toured India,

*However, aware of the difficulties non-Hindus encounter with the correct pronunciation of *mantras* (phonemes derived from the fifty letters of the Sanskrit alphabet), Sri Goswami, pure teacher that he was, confined his teaching of Laya Yoga in the West to theory only.

the United States, Japan, and several European countries, during which he presented conferences that were illustrated with demonstrations of Haṭha Yoga.

In 1949, Shyam Sundar Goswami represented India in the World Physical Education Congress in Lingiaden, Sweden. During the course of this international meeting a delegation of doctors, filled with enthusiasm for his demonstrations of physiological control that had previously been considered impossible, asked him to found an institute in Stockholm. From that point on, he tirelessly taught the theory and practices of Yoga. The Goswami Yoga Institute, which is probably the oldest Yoga school in Europe, contributed to the spread and revival of this discipline in Western countries.

At the time of his visit to Paris, from late 1950 to early 1951, the greatest medical institutions (Salpêtrière, Assistance Publique des Hôpitaux de Paris), cultural organizations (the Guimet Museum, UNESCO), and the press paid tribute to his conferences and demonstrations. On account of his erudition and his rare skill at transmitting, in scientific terms, the message of Yoga, Shyam Sundar Goswami came to be internationally recognized by his peers as a master.

Remarkable achievements may be put to his credit, such as the introduction to the West of both the full control of the rectus abdominis and that of the smooth musculature (Naulī). The latter was clinically presented to a baffled medical audience with the demonstration of rare urethral suctions of air, water, and milk respectively. Educational credit should also be awarded to the Goswami Yoga Institute for having shown in a university physiology clinic the possibility for human beings to sustain hyperventilation at a speed level above 220 respirations per minute, continually and for more than one hour. This was done at a time when Western lung physiology manuals stated the rate of 100 respirations per minute as the maximum voluntary hyperventilation.

This Yoga pioneer died in Stockholm on October 13, 1978, at the age of eighty-seven. Today there remains of this life—which included seventy uninterrupted years devoted to the study, exercise, and teaching of the vast subject of Yoga—two works considered as classics of yogic literature, *Advanced Haṭha Yoga* (Inner Traditions, 2012) and *Layayoga*

(Inner Traditions, 1999), as well as a significant number of new manuscripts, including the proceedings of a hundred selected conferences translated into French, Swedish, and Kurdish. A selected number of his lectures are now available on the website dedicated to this great son of spiritual India (www.goswamiyogainstitute.com).

Shyam Sundar Goswami remains little known in the English-speaking world. This book, which aims to make a modest contribution to the understanding of this Yoga master and his teaching, is the first book in the English language that is entirely devoted to him.

My Meeting with a Yoga Master

My first meeting with Sri Shyam Sundar Goswami took place one fine autumn day during a conference given by this cultivated globetrotter at Konserthuset, in Stockholm, Sweden.

It was only later that I understood the truly remarkable nature of our encounter, which took place on September 7, 1956—an auspicious day, since it was my birthday. Moreover, that very morning my son was born, the first child of a happy marriage. My initial relationship with this yogi was only the formal one of teacher to pupil, but in time it would develop into something different.

From my early youth, I had already been interested in philosophy. One day I was chauffeuring the "Professor"—the title used by his Swedish entourage—and I asked him the meaning of two Sanskrit terms that I had gleaned from reading an oriental text. Rarely a loquacious person, the passenger of my little Citroën car replied: "If you really want to know the answer, you should come to my Raja Yoga classes."

Despite family obligations, financial constraints, and the handicap that was placed on me by being an immigrant worker, my thirst for knowledge was so great that I attended his classes. At first, I inevitably suffered from a lack of comprehension of the numerous technical terms, both in English and Sanskrit, that came out of the mouth of this modern St. John Chrysostom, a man of exceptional erudition.

At the beginning of our relationship, the Professor was, in my eyes, just a brilliant representative of Indian culture who was involved in learned research. But after a certain amount of hesitation on my part, arising from my innate skepticism, Sri S. S. Goswami would become for me not only the transmitter of a vast body of knowledge relating to every aspect of life, but also what Hindus from all castes and epochs call a guru—a spiritual guide.

So it came to pass that I had the privilege not only of studying, practicing, and experiencing the discipline of Yoga under his direction, but also of enriching all my intellectual perspectives and awakening my latent spirituality. After a while, I even had the remarkable honor of assisting him in his daily affairs.

It was only after two decades of continual study and practice that this founding father of modern Yoga, a short while before his death, deemed it appropriate to grant me a formal initiation (*dīkṣā*) that would perpetuate the extraordinary Guru Yoga relationship of teacher and disciple, the unfailing presence of a guide, friend, and counselor. It was a relationship that allowed me to discover myself, while leaving me free to appreciate the beauty of friendship and pure love, which is the essence of all manifested spirituality. It was not until several years later, during a journey in India, that Ma Santi Devi, his spiritual mother, offered me the final initiation granted to yogis by traditional Yoga—a rare occurrence for a Westerner—just as she had done for Sri Goswami, her most illustrious disciple. Thus did she invite me to follow to the best of my ability the teachings of this exiled Bengali master, and so included me in a spiritual lineage dating back at least seven centuries.

To this brief testimonial I add those of several other people who, like me, had the opportunity to cross paths with Shyam Sundar Goswami. Professor Gunnar Adler-Karlsson (student of the Nobel Prize–winning economist, Gunnar Myrdal) wrote: "From the bottom of my heart, I express my gratitude to this glorious soul. . . . He was an example of one who concentrated on what was essential—life itself. . . . In his presence, it was out of the question to lie or to deviate from the absolute truth. . . . His sense of morality towered above that of anyone else I have known; he was a brilliant example of right conduct. . . . I would have been unable to overcome my difficulties without the strength that I received from his serenity and the love of truth that he taught me."

Sri Karunamoya Saraswati, one of India's four experts (*ācāryas*) on Hindu scriptures in the 1940s, stated: "Shyam Sundar Goswami is the greatest interpreter of Yoga in modern times."

Dr. Ulf Jansson, a medical doctor and close pupil who was particularly interested in the anatomy of the chakras, declared that "the 'Professor' [Goswami] was animated by a true passion for scientific investigation, and the systematization of his subject of research. . . . I have always been able to count on him, even in the midst of a crisis or illness; always attentive, he listened to me relating my problems and offered me his enlightened advice and often the hospitality of his table. Each time that I visited him, I was transported into a great hope for the future, into an intense feeling of joy and happiness."

Claude Kayat, author of several nominated novels, said that "he was a prodigious monument to strength, and we sat at his feet eager to learn. . . . In retrospect, I realized that it was without doubt those times, seated on a blanket spread out on his rug, that I experienced the most precious moments of my life."

For Ingjald Starråker, chief editor of *Utrikespolitiska Institutet:*

> Goswami was a remarkable person. Most striking in him, I found, was fidelity to truth. He never claimed faculties he didn't possess or to have done things he didn't do. He was fully free from any trace of false modesty, which is a modified form of a lie. His opinions on other people could be very sharp but his descriptions most pertinent. One could always trust him.

Vishuddhananda Giri, his would-be disciple and spiritual heir, felt: "His whole personality inspired equally the ideal of yogic excellence (*deva deha*) and the ideas of Ancient Greece: strength, wisdom, courage, and beauty—what we call life. . . . During the whole of my long life, he was a master, counselor, and friend—a guru, a spiritual father."

Finally, Julia Martinez, a dedicated pupil of the Goswami Yoga Institute, says she is "faithful in my heart to the grace of having touched those who met him."

Sri Goswami's Yoga Teaching

It is not always easy with Sri Shyam Sundar Goswami to distinguish the teaching from the teacher, to understand someone who dispenses knowledge and wisdom in measured doses and, amid his own students, is a living example of the metaphysical synthesis of all knowledge. This is why, before looking at his teachings, it is perhaps instructive for the reader to enter into the world inhabited by this exceptional being, whose cognitive ethical fabric was most intriguing.

From the outset, a person visiting this Hindu sage would be impressed by the silence and the tranquil atmosphere that reigned in his study, which was filled with an impressive quantity of books and manuscripts and was located in his rented modest apartment in a quiet neighborhood of the Swedish capital.

The visitor would first see him from the back, seated in his armchair, his upper body always absolutely straight, his build athletic, and a shock of white hair crowning his tilted head. The scratching sound of a Parker pen would give away the fact that he was writing on one of the lined pages in his notebook.

At the beginning of his stay in Sweden, Sri Goswami gave three theory lessons a week, reduced later to two lessons when he began organizing his biweekly coed practical classes. His lessons followed faithfully the rhythm of university courses, with two breaks, one in the summer and the other at the end of the year. The theme of each of these biweekly lessons was different and they continued in parallel throughout the year. He always approached the subjects under discussion in a methodical and scientifically rigorous manner. His discourses, which were for the most part instructional, were sprinkled with anecdotes, digressions, or comparisons arising from recent discoveries in the fields of neurology or nuclear physics.

He could be impenetrable and even appear obscure; sometimes the new perspectives he suggested were highly thought provoking, and sometimes the depth or originality of the concept he introduced was baffling. The teacher's language was always articulate and allowed moments of silence in which to choose the perfect word. With a respectful audience—in spite of his arguments or assertions that could at first glance sometimes appear iconoclastic to scientists or professors of medicine—he also made room for a request for clarification, unless it was a question of satisfying a typist who was anxious to transcribe a Sanskrit term accurately.

Sri S. S. Goswami's courses included the central themes of human sciences, and, while sounding scientific when he interpreted Hindu metaphysics or spiritual experiences, he gave equal consideration to physical education, diet, advanced hygiene, fasting, mastery of the mind, the application of Yoga's ethical rules, and erudite commentaries on classical Hindu writings. He could easily switch from sharing advanced expositions to making theories concrete when imparting private instructions. There he displayed a yogic know-how that could only have seen the light of day through his own practice and numerous experiences.

Always rational, his teaching was able to take into account the recurring problem for every Westerner: remaining seated with legs crossed and the back perfectly straight and immobile, which is a basic posture for the fundamental exercise of mental concentration.

Sri Goswami did not hesitate to reveal the oral tradition of *cāraṇā,* an ancient form of yogic bodybuilding that remains undocumented to this day. The secret of this method of physical education is still jealously guarded by its practitioners, notably those yogis who appear only every four years, on the occasion of traditional *kumba melas*—popular gatherings that are much esteemed in Indian spirituality.

In addition to the importance of diet and the necessity of physical training suited to modern life, Sri Goswami emphasized the importance of good elimination of intestinal waste, something that is too often neglected in our sedentary societies. Peerless teacher that he was, he insisted moreover on the necessity of remembering, as part of one's Yoga plan, to maintain optimal vitality in the organs, which results in the retardation of the undesirable effects of aging.

During two world tours, Professor Shyam Sundar Goswami introduced the discipline of Yoga in scientific terms, thus building a lasting bridge between India and the West. Wherever he lectured (primarily medical establishments), accompanied by his close student, Dr. D. Pramanick, he gave demonstrations of muscle and organ control, which until then had been considered impossible. These demonstrations elicited considerable interest in the United States as well as in Europe.

He knew how to extract and present to modern humans an understandable and practical version of the ancient science of Yoga, purged of all ritual (*puja* and *bajan*) or religion, while maintaining great respect for the spiritual sensitivities of his new followers. As a result, in the years following World War II, a doctrine that had often been considered abstruse was transmitted in terms that were understandable in spite of inherent cultural differences. Often faced with many challenges in translating Sanskrit terms, the Indian master drew from books on anatomy, human physiology, neurology, or physics in order to make himself correctly understood. Gifted with a brilliant mind, which was both methodical and creative, he never hesitated to enrich the language of Yoga with neologisms when he wished to describe profound potentialities.

Retaining the pragmatism that characterizes the nature of a thinker and a man of action, while remaining faithful to the tradition of Yoga, Sri S. S. Goswami's teaching was essentially oriented toward a mastery of the mind and the body, which led the adept to the sublime yogic ideal of *deva deha* (outstanding being). His teaching included the basic subject matters that relate to the study of the fundamental questions of our existence: human ontology, eschatology, with (in the context of Hinduism) the underlying theory of rebirth, as well as yogic salvation, which is traditionally a theistic liberation.

This Yoga master taught at three related but distinct levels, according to the leanings and maturity of the pupil. For certain students, renewed physical and mental well-being were their primary motivation; for others, it was the philosophical aspect of the discourse that awakened their intellectual curiosity. In a restricted circle of ambitious pupils, these two complementary aspects were not sufficient; such students needed the fulfillment of profound study, probing into the mysteries of the mind. For others, religious feeling stimulated an unquestioning adherence to the spiritual ideal presented by this remarkable representative of Yoga; although they remained true to their own beliefs, they asked him to assume the role of their spiritual guide.

A summary of the lessons of this master of Hindu wisdom would involve recalling the pains he took to emphasize the link Yoga created between science and philosophy, remembering his exposition of an ancient culture that in fact constitutes the incontrovertible essence of every religion, and his guidance not to consider human beings solely in the light of their qualities, virtues, apparent limitations, ethnic origin, social standing, or any aspect of their personality whatsoever. From this broad perspective, an integrated person who is aware of our potential and true nature, beyond the acknowledged infinities of microphysics and astrophysics, must evolve in all the conscious levels of being: the body, *prāna* (vital life force), mind (meaning here the intellect, will, feeling, and aesthetic sense), morality, religion, and the spiritual life.

From this enlarged point of view, a human declares himself or herself a being of both reflection and action, accepting the duty not only to succeed in one's own life, but also to exhibit compassion, altruism, determination, and faith. A lover of truth, such a person is magnanimous and capable of abandoning personal convictions in favor of those that surpass them. In this way a person can free himself or herself of the prejudices and limitations that block a transcendent realization of Self.

It is to Sri Shyam Sundar Goswami that the reader should attribute the merit of the truths set out in this work, and only to his disciple should blame be addressed for any errors from which the text suffers.

1
Origins and Objectives of Yoga

The origin of Yoga goes back to the period of Vedic civilization, probably five thousand years before Jesus Christ. Nevertheless, rock inscriptions in the form of yogic postures discovered in 1952 at Addaura, on Sicily, seem to bear witness to the presence of *āsanas* (yogic postures) in the Mediterranean between 10,000 and 15,000 BCE. More recent remains in India, dating from 2475 to 3000 BCE, attest to the fact that yogic postures were known there during the Vedic period. Discoveries made in Mohenjo-Daro, in modern-day Pakistan, confirm this theory.

Reflections on the Sacred Texts of India

The sages of India consider the Vedas and the Tantras to be the two arms of the divine power supporting the universe. Dating back to time immemorial, emerging out of India's prehistory, and the source of numerous sacred texts, the Vedas are not of human origin. They are neither the fruit of intellectual speculation nor the expression of dogmatic or ritualistic beliefs. Symbolically, they emanate from the mouth of Brahmā, one of the three Hindu gods. The Tantras, on the other hand,

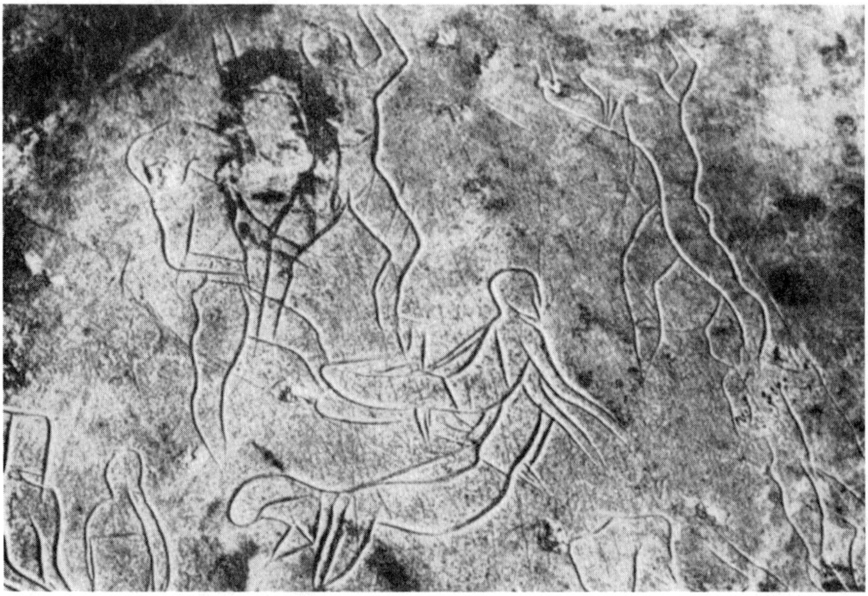

Fig. 1.1. The Addaura Cave on Sicily

which are almost as ancient, come from Śiva, the god of destruction and reproduction.

The Vedas, source of all Yoga, were "seen" by Brahmā, the first rishi and Yoga guru. The different aspects of Vedic Yoga were then explained by Viṣṇu, while Śiva, often regarded as the actual father of Yoga, gave it a new and detailed interpretation. Vedic Yoga was collected in the Tantras to become Tantric Yoga. The original Vedic exposition of Yoga is thus detailed in the Upaniṣads, while Tantric Yoga is fully explained in the Tantras. The rishis' various interpretations of Yoga have been collected in the Itihāsas and the Purāṇas. Advanced understanding of Yoga therefore is conveyed via a study of the Vedas. The term *Yoga* is mentioned in the *Mantra Veda,* while its essence is integrated into the Gāyatrī Mantra of the *Ṛigveda.*

The complete experience of the Vedas is a revelation of all possible knowledge. In theological terms, it corresponds to the experience of the omniscience of Brahmā. The Vedas therefore contain the quintessence of all scientific and spiritual knowledge, every area of wisdom accessible to humans:

1. Ultimate knowledge of the Supreme Being (*asamprajñāta samādhi*)
2. Supraconscious knowledge of the Supreme Being and of objects at different levels (*samprajñāta samādhi*)
3. Cognitive realizations at the suprasensory level (*dhyāna*)
4. Superior intellectual knowledge of spiritual and physical sciences
5. Knowledge of all sensory perceptions

Tradition refers to the Vedas as *śruti,* a term that implies a sound or visual revelation perceived in a transcendental state of mental concentration (*dhyāna* or *samādhi*). According to this same tradition, all existing truth can be revealed to anyone empowered to receive it. This obviously doesn't mean that a person who can hear or see a truth thus revealed is the creator or the inventor of it. The genius of a Newton or an Einstein does not make these scientists respectively the creators of gravitation or cosmic relativity. They can only claim to have discovered and enunciated the mechanisms that govern these two physical phenomena. Similarly, in their supraconscious vision (*dhi*) of the Vedas, the rishis or seers received a limited understanding of the elements of life, the mind, and matter.

A gigantic magnum opus of a billion verses, the Vedas were revised by the sage Vyāsa,* who abbreviated them in eighteen parts amounting to four hundred thousand verses. The texts of the Brāhmaṇas, which were taken from the original Vedas and are assumed to be encyclopedic, were written by the rishis from the Vedic *mantras,* written components of the Samhītās (collection of scriptures) of the Vedas. The Brāhmaṇas facilitate the comprehension of the Vedas. They cover subjects related to social or political matters as well as the religions of ancient India.

The Brāhmaṇic scriptures are also made up of the Upaniṣads, of which 108 are available today. These scriptures explain Yoga and the way of obtaining a state of supreme consciousness that corresponds to the direct realization of the Absolute (Brahman). They explain the

*Vyāsa was the Indian sage who is also considered the author of great Hindu epics, notably the famous *Mahābhārata.*

nature of the mind as well as the pranic forces or the *nāḍīs* that are traces of subtle kinetic currents.*

There are several further studies on the scriptures called the Smṛiti Samhītās, which deal mainly with questions of law, traditions and customs, and codes of behavior. Also of note is a discourse on the practice of divine love, of which the most known presentation is that of Angira, entitled *Daiva Mīmāmsādarśana.*

We should also mention the six *darśanas.* In the absence of an equivalent term, *darśana* is most often translated as "philosophy," although, strictly speaking, it means "point of view." A better translation might be "paradigm demonstration," in the epistemological sense of the word. *Darśana* suggests the direct experience of the physical, mental, and spiritual world, as well as the acquisition of knowledge by research, study, experiment, and intuition. Of the six "points of view"—that is to say, the *Vaiśeṣikadarśana* of Kanada, the *Nyāyadarśana* of Gautama, the *Samkyadarśana* of Kapila, the *Pūrva Mīmāmsādarśana* of Jaimini, the *Vedāntadarśana* of Vyāsa, and the *Yogadarśana* of Patañjali†—the *Yogadarśana* is undoubtedly the most widespread in the West. The aphorisms of Patañjali's classical work, dedicated to the study and practice of Yoga, were introduced into Europe by the German philosopher Schopenhauer in the nineteenth century.

The attempt to date the Vedas has led to many hypotheses by various erudite people. They refer on the one hand to the rich oral tradition and to the exegesis of Hindu scriptures, and on the other hand to conclusions (often hasty and conjectural) based mainly on archaeological excavations. The Western conception of time is generally limited to paleontological and archaeological discoveries, which define our history as dating back eight thousand years. However, cosmological conclusions in India open up much vaster horizons.

These ideas would seem purely fictitious were it not for the fact that we have long been aware of the innovative role of Indian culture

*It is tempting to assimilate these intangibles into the theory of strings and superstrings that aims to reconcile general relativity and quantum mechanics.

†Patañjali was an Indian philosopher and grammarian (around the second century BCE).

in many domains, notably in arithmetic and astronomy. For example, one could quote the rishi Kanada, whose ideas foreshadowed atomic theory and considered light and heat as two forms of the same primordial substance. Incidentally, it is the same Kanada whose description of Kuṇḍalinī as Supreme Power, with reference to his global vision proclaims that it "shines like ten million suns and is bright and cool like ten million moons and splendorous like lightning" (*Tārārahasya*).

Is the teaching of Indian sacred texts really more disturbing than that of recent astrophysical and subatomic advances, which for approximately the last two centuries have tirelessly expanded the limits of the universe and its contents? In the West physical science has made great progress since the time of Democritus, the first man in history to put forward a theory of atoms, and even more progress since Heraclitus, who considered the universe to be an incessantly moving world and was thus in direct opposition to the spiritual father of contemporary science, Parmenides of Elea. Known by Plato as the "Great One," Parmenides' holistic understanding of "being is what is, nonbeing is what is not" was singularly close to Vedic monism.

Many erudite paradigms have been introduced since Aristotle placed the earth in the middle of the universe and since the emancipating revolution of Copernicus, who allowed our Western ancestors, ignorant or neglectful of the rest of the universe, to break the planetary preeminence in which they believed they lived.

Moreover, what can be said about the recent increase in the total number of known galaxies—mapped to an astonishing 260 thousand—other than it abolishes the myth of a solar system that enjoys a unique status? And what can be said of the dizzying idea put forward by today's scientists of an expanding flat universe, evolving cyclically, with a diameter of 1,600,000,000 km, which, since the last cataclysm, would be several billion years old? Or, in an increasingly surprising "multiverse" revealed by NASA's recent and equally amazing study, indicating that our own galaxy gives shelter to 46 billion planets with sizes that are similar to that of our planet Earth?

What can we expect from research into a truth that, in the light of these recent discoveries, has drifted into the notion of a macrocosm that seems to be fused with the microcosm? Do not the potential variants of the theory of strings and superstrings, which aim to reconcile general relativity and quantum mechanics, open new perspectives on the current instrument-based research, which is imprisoned in the four human dimensions—three spatial and one temporal—a limitation that forever prohibits access into a universe composed of ten or eleven dimensions, if not more? A pragmatic mind will suggest that all these facts, proven or supposed, cannot really disturb the familiar oasis of which an ordinary person's life consists.

The wisdom of Indian holy writings is not the expression of an intellectual ideology that refutes all reality and the world. Nor is it, moreover, the reflection of an anthropogenic principle that would not concede any particular interest to the universe except to its materially observable aspects.

In the vision of the rishis, time is eternal. That is to say, time is without end, consisting of a past with no beginning and a future with no end. The creation of the cosmos is a repetitive, tangible manifestation of the Absolute. In the succession of cycles (*manvantara**), time consists of the inseparable phenomena of creation and destruction that characterize cosmic evolution. Each cycle is endowed with a cosmic progenitor (Manu). In the current era (*yuga*) he is called Vaivasvata. In his role as the prototype of humanity, this progenitor corresponds approximately to the Hebrew tradition of Adam.

Probably inspired by Hermes Trismegistus, who asserted in the *Book of the Twenty-four Philosophers* that "God is an infinite sphere, the center of which is everywhere, the circumference nowhere," Pascal, and probably many others with him, duplicated that concept, but substituted the universe for God at the center of their thesis and declared: "The universe is an infinite sphere, the center of which is everywhere, the circumference nowhere."

Hindu cosmology postulates the existence of an underlying static, causal principle endowed with the power to "will" and to express the dynamic aspect of a static eternal reality. Following this view, whatever

*Concerning the chronological reality of the duration of *manvantara*, read notably René Guénon, *Formes traditionnelles et cycles cosmiques* (Gallimard, 1970).

manifests in the cosmos constitutes the circumference that is everywhere, while the center (the unmanifested) upon which it depends is nowhere. In this paradigm, one motionless Prime mover is the origin of all cosmic manifestation and its amazing biodiversity and changes.

The dissolution of the cosmos coincides with the beginning of a period of nonmanifestation, which, in symbolic terms, is neither more nor less than a return to the supreme source—Brahman, or the Absolute. Out of this Absolute a new manifestation then emerges. This alternation is described allegorically as "the days and nights of Brahmā." According to recent interpretations of ancient writings, notably the *Śrīmad Bhāgavatam,* the duration of "a day of Brahmā," or *kalpa,* is determined with a degree of arithmetical precision: the philosopher O. V. Krishnamurthy asserts that this duration, which cannot be conceived by thought, is 4,320 million years. These esoteric calculations divide space-time into fourteen periods (*manvantara*) and seventy-one ultimate subdivisions (Mahā Yuga), each one consisting of four phases: Satya Yuga, Treta Yuga, Dvapara Yuga, and lastly Kali Yuga, the current period, which will last 432 thousand years, which, in symbolic terms, is neither more nor less than a return to the supreme source—Brahman, or the Absolute, the thrice great (*sat cit ānanda*).

In ancient Greece and Rome, this cosmological order corresponded to the ages of gold, silver, bronze, and iron, glorified by, among others, the poet Virgil:

> *Once more the great order of the centuries begins.*
> *Already a new race is descending from the lofty sky.*
> *Then the golden race will appear for the entire world.*

As with the *kalpa,* this unimaginable "day of Brahmā," which comes after the passing of a cosmic night, is followed by a corresponding period. Brahmā is himself followed by another Brahmā in an infinite cycle, once again inconceivable for the human imagination. . . .

At the frontier of experimental science, a number of important contemporary scientists glimpse another reality than that which is accessible today. Thus does the physicist Schrödinger, author of several philosophical works and an adept of the monist doctrine, invoke the Vedas in order to explain his concept of the world. For his part, Ilya Prigogine, Nobel Laureate for Chemistry in 1997, mentions "the possibility of an eternal recommencement of an infinite series of universes."*

In the book by Fred Alan Wolf, *Taking the Quantum Leap* (Harper and Row, 1989). Richard Phillips Feynman, one of the most influential physicists of the last century, compares the subtle mechanisms of our individuality to an atomic dance similar to the cosmic dance of Śiva: "Atoms enter my brain, perform a dance, and then they exit; forever new atoms, but forever the same dance." The same thing is said by Fritjof Capra, a philosopher and theoretical physicist, in his preface to *The Tao of Physics* (Shambhala, 1975).

In a scientific study by Sir Roger Penrose, *Cycles of Time: An Extraordinary New View of the Universe,* the author certainly did not disappoint his learned peers regarding the "extraordinary": he describes the unfathomable origins of a cyclic cosmos by asserting that "the Big Bang is both the end of one eon and the beginning of another."

At the risk of giving superficial consideration to a subject many Western and other researchers have investigated for decades, it seems necessary to briefly review the controversy that exists in an academic world that favors theory over pragmatic research and logic over intuitive introspection.

It is not improbable that the Vedas, which are the first known writings, are much older than the age proposed by Western researchers, who too often demonstrate condescension instead of humility and a priori approaches rather than the objectivity that is the responsibility of the scientific mind. In this way their claimed objectivity has suffered from various handicaps: adherence to a religion supposed to have the monopoly on truth; privileged participation in a culture known for its technological prowess; adherence to a society that has bet on material progress for its salvation; inheritance of a civilization with a glorious past and, believing itself superior in every respect, possessed by the mission to conquer and dominate.

*In Ilya Prigogine and Isabelle Sengers, *Entre le Temps et l'Éternité* (Fayard, 1988).

It is regrettable that too often the objectivity of Western intellectuals has been unable to take into account the influence of Hindu thought, though it has been well documented, in particular by the philosophers of Ancient Greece, the so-called cradle of Western civilization.

We have been given due warning about this inappropriate feeling of superiority in many ways, including through the false interpretation of the Sanskrit term *āryan* (virtuous, noble) by Max Müller.* In 1853, this German orientalist introduced the term into the West to designate a particular race and its language. Faced with lively criticism from contemporary intellectuals and historians, Max Müller was forced several years later to do his mea culpa for his thesis, the interpretation of which, though not intentionally, carried in its bosom the seed of a regrettably grievous racism. But it was too late, the evil was done, and, like any calumny that can never truly be effaced, the thesis of an Aryan race rapidly took root in several countries, in particular in the heart of German nationalism, which found in it an opportunity to promote its ideology of white supremacy. This ended in the barbarism we know about, the immolation of several million human beings.

Another reason for the depreciation of Hindu civilization resides in the theory of a supposed Aryan invasion of Sanskrit-speaking "Indo-European" northerners via Central Asia. Between 1500 and 1200 BCE these white-skinned peoples are supposed to have invaded an India that was then inhabited essentially by Dravidians and groups of people from the Indian southern peninsula who had brown skins and were considered inferior. The theory of an invasion by Aryan Vedic people seems to present the only serious proof in a doubtful or malevolent interpretation of certain Hindu writings, notably the *Ṛigveda*. However, this text refers in fact to a racial mixture instead of what one would expect—a description of an alleged struggle of light-skinned against dark-skinned people. This is a strange assertion if one considers that this same *Ṛigveda* indicates that birth cannot be considered as identifying one who is "Aryan"!†

*German linguist (1823–1900), author of numerous studies on the religions of India.

†In *The Myth of the Aryan Invasion of India* (South Asia Books, 1994), the eminent Dr. David Frawley, expert in the Vedas (vedācārya), sets out edifying conclusions on the subject.

The theory of an Aryan invasion seems to crumble following recent archaeological discoveries and cartography, established with the aid of satellites, of the Saraswati River. These evidence the continuity of the Vedic and Saraswati civilizations. In India, the absurdity of the hypothesis of an Aryan invasion has been set out by a particular circumstance, invoked by great thinkers such as Jandhyala B. G. Tilak, Dayananda Saraswati, as well as one of the great names in contemporary spiritual thought, Sri Aurobindo. According to the Vedic writings they invoke, the supposed Aryan invaders mention the names of no religious sites outside of India; they only glorify existing religious sites like the Ganges River, Varanasi, and so on.

Max Müller's thesis, according to which the birth of the Vedic culture dates back to 1500 BCE, thus collapses. According to many intellectuals in India, the date would instead be between twelve thousand and eight thousand years before the Greco-Roman world and the era of Christianity. As a result, is it not plausible to affirm that the ideological justification of the British invasion of the Indian continent, as well as the cultural North-South tensions that would later follow in India, are without doubt the fruit of these false interpretations? Moreover, we can only deplore the *tamasic* (inertial) passivity of the Brahmin scholars who adhere, in overwhelming silence or guilty complicity, to these mistaken ideas and thus endorse hasty and irresponsible conclusions drawn from a disastrous theory.

We should also say a few words about the term *Hinduism,* which is linked to a Vedic civilization several millennia old that ran through a complex kaleidoscope of historical, cultural, and spiritual expressions. Although Hinduism is effectively a religion in the conventional sense of the term—that is to say with texts, rituals, and a moral code—it nevertheless distinguishes itself by its immanence, fluidity, resilience, and rare faculty of absorbing all religious dogmas (is there not a work entitled *Allah Upaniṣad*?). At the risk of sometimes being accused of an extreme tolerance in its timeless aspiration to universality, it is *sanātana dharma,* the eternal charioteer of the Bhagavad Gītā, the imperishable theme of Hindu thought.

Hinduism is then characterized by a conceptual epistemology, which, paradoxically as it may seem to the Western mind, embraces at the same time the dual and the nondual, along with other seemingly contradictory aspects: monotheistic in proclaiming the One-and-All doctrine; polytheistic when venerating 300 million deities; pantheistic when identifying Brahman with the universe; and, indeed, atheistic when the *jīvanmukta,* or "liberated alive," witnesses an ultimate transcending experience of *mokṣa,* the merger between *ātman* and *paramātman,* the indescribable Absolute sometimes referred to as That.

Hinduism's attraction for free-thinking, non-Hindu born people is often explained by the absence of dogma and its extreme tolerance, not just a conventional tolerance but an actual respect for all faiths. At the socioreligious level Hinduism proposes a deeper and broader understanding of traditional religious teachings, which at the individual level is reflected by pragmatic approaches that include the inborn dynamism and dormant faculties of the human being. In the daily perception of such an all-embracing vision lies the real source for brotherhood, mutual respect, and natural impulses to help the needy. In daily life's dilemma of opposed opinions, it successfully brings forth solutions in a holistic paradigm that applies the unwritten principle of complementarity.

Given the complexity of Hinduism, the oldest of all religions, what is surprising to researchers concerned about objectivity, as well as to historians, anthropologists, and theologians, is Hinduism's unequalled continuity of a sociocultural dynamic, an uninterrupted current with a multitude of ever-changing facets. Rather than propose a servile submission to clerical authority, which not only has no actual possibility of verifying mystical experience but may even find it embarrassing or threatening to its temporal power, the Hindu spiritual quest has no other aspiration than to discover our true identity and to attain liberation from attachment to the illusion of our human condition. Embarking on a spiritual path that does not ignore the misery of the world in which we live, the spiritual seeker begins a quest of becoming acquainted with the experience of yogis and rishis—those exceptional beings who in all times have known how to successfully tackle the possibility of union and supreme bliss with the Divine, which is the ultimate goal of human destiny.

The Yogic Path

In this period of the widespread rediscovery of Yoga, and of Haṭha Yoga in particular, it seems desirable to present briefly and in contemporary terms the tenets and objectives of the yogic path, which offers a vast source of knowledge that constantly has new applications in today's changing world.

Traditional texts of India present Yoga as the ultimate human attainment. They also explain the exact way of reaching the state of a yogi, the attainment of a primordial consciousness that prepares the way for union with God. Here it is important to keep in mind that the notion of God conveyed by Indian sacred writings differs from that of the Judeo-Christian world. In fact, the term *God* does not exist in the sacred writings of India, although a multitude of names are given for multiple aspects of God. To avoid misunderstanding, however, we can consider the word *God* in the Hindu sense as an approximation of what is generally understood in the contemporary Western world.

This same tradition attributes the origin of Yoga to the god Śiva. Originally called Mahā Yoga, it gave rise to a hundred paths of Yoga. The elaboration given by the Upaniṣads concerning the eightfold path of Yoga (Aṣṭānga Yoga) permitted the emergence of new methods and techniques, which are differentiated into two fundamental aspects: the acquisition of powers and the spiritual realization of the individual. In his research, Sri Goswami identified a large number of Yoga variations, some distinct and some similar: twenty-four in the Upaniṣads, forty-three in the Tantras, four in the *Yogavasiṣṭa,* two in the *Rāmāyana,* thirty-one in the *Mahābhārata,* and two hundred and twelve in the Purāṇas.

Of these, only four have survived to this day: Mantra Yoga, Haṭ ha Yoga, Laya Yoga (or Kuṇḍalinī Yoga), and Raja Yoga. The last of these, commonly named the "Royal Way," is related to other paths such as the Yoga of Knowledge (Jñāna Yoga), the Yoga of Devotion to the Divine (Bhakti Yoga), Yoga of Action (Karma Yoga), and many more. Śiva is credited with the following remark on the complementary role of the two principal paths of Yoga: "Without the practice of Raja Yoga, Haṭha Yoga remains incomplete. Without Haṭha Yoga, the practice of Raja Yoga is impossible."

The way of Haṭha Yoga is both a traditional path of pragmatic spiritual research and a nearly inexhaustible source of human knowledge—a "science of man." As such, the all-embracing discipline of Haṭha Yoga is a most adequate and versatile "Middle Way" lifestyle, where anyone may faithfully comply with life's obligations and pleasures while still participating in the spiritual quest of Yoga *sādhana* (practice).

Inspired by the holistic scheme of life set forth in the Bhagavad

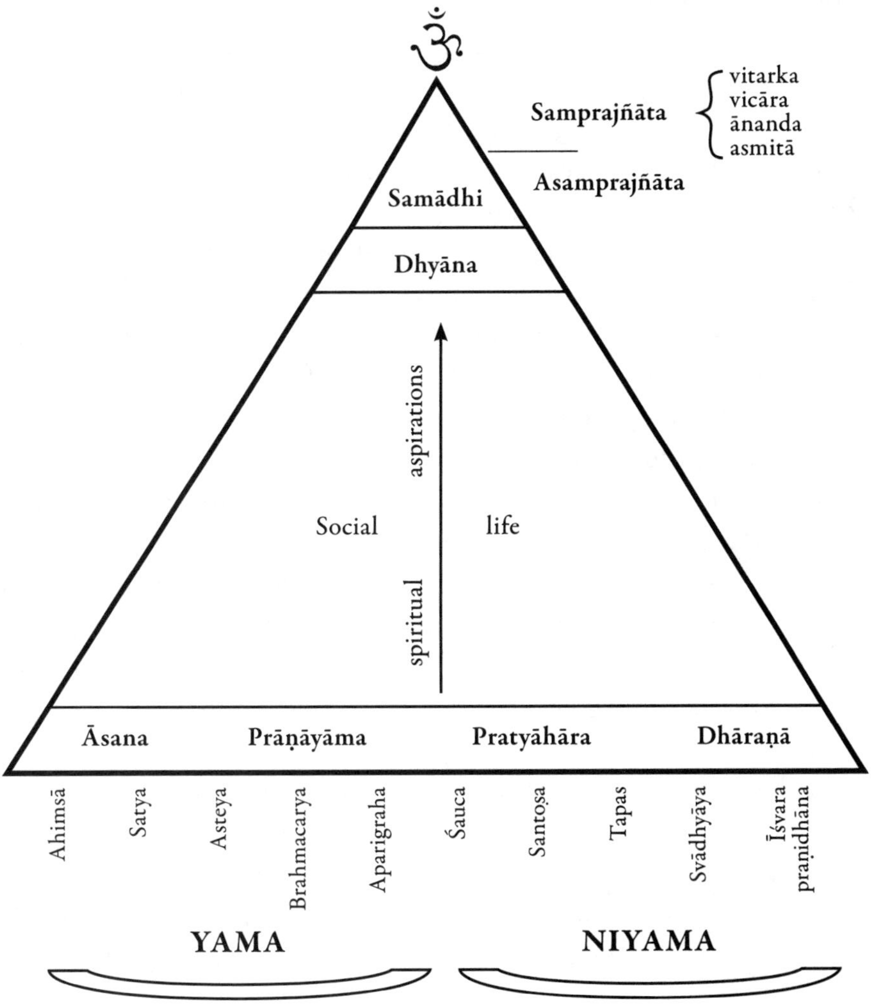

Fig. 1.2. In the Middle Way *sādhana*, spiritual aspirations help a person to weather the ups and downs of social life, guided by the ethical rules of *yama* and *niyama*, which are the essence of all sincere spiritual search.

Gītā's triptych of knowledge, action, and love, and following Tantra's rational philosophy, the Middle Way lifestyle aims at bringing together opposites and, ultimately, transcendentally merging into a sublime state of existence-nonexistence. This ontological proposal challenges the Shakespearian dilemma "To be or not to be." It affirms the sublime option of: "To be *and* not to be"!

Haṭha Yoga not only allows a person to find inner peace and to reshape and master the body; it also shapes the senses and the mind into an instrument capable of discovering states of consciousness located beyond the sensory world. It can also provide the means to attain a spiritual peak that is nothing less than the realization of an immanent and transcendent truth, a supreme union, a goal that is characteristic of all forms of living spirituality. In the Hindu tradition, Yoga—with its elements, metaphysics, purifications, and palette of methods—constitutes the bridge that links the human to the Divine.

In the Northern hemisphere, it is above all the *āsanas* or postures of Haṭha Yoga that retain our attention, most often in the harmless form of physical training, relaxation, sport, or as a therapeutic method, with the limited goal of achieving physical well-being or regaining psychological equilibrium. In truth, though the traditional goal of the psychophysical exercises includes the aims of any physical activity (suppleness, strength, speed, and endurance), Haṭha Yoga offers other advantages such as durable peace of mind, the sense of harmony resulting from awareness of the body, mastery of the breath, and enhancement of mental concentration, which is the essential foundation for mastery of the mind.

It is important to remember that *āsanas* are only one of eight parts of Haṭha Yoga. Though it is true that this discipline attaches great importance to the body, which is the keystone of our mental and spiritual life, nevertheless this is only one step in the eightfold path considered as sacred. These eight disciplines, which we will consider later in more detail, are:

1. *Yama*—five ethical rules: *ahimsā, satya, asteya, brahmacarya, aparigraha*

2. *Niyama*—five additional rules: *śauca, santoṣa, tapas, svādhyāya, īśvarapraṇidhāna*
3. *Āsana*—psychophysical exercises
4. *Prāṇāyāma*—mastery of *prāṇa* (breath as life force)
5. *Pratyāhāra*—mental process of withdrawing from sensory objects
6. *Dhāraṇā*—first step of mental concentration
7. *Dhyāna*—second step of mental concentration
8. *Samādhi*—apogee of mental concentration

With its eight disciplines, Haṭha Yoga thus constitutes a form of the very ancient Aṣṭānga Yoga, which deals with human beings in all their aspects, manifest and latent, gross and subtle—or, in other words, in all the aspects of our physical, vital, and mental life, including our behavior, will, affective life, and spirituality. Haṭha Yoga also presents unique purification techniques that permit the attainment of an optimal state of purity, toning of the vital force, and improvement of the faculty of perception.

The aim of Yoga, which represents the ultimate exploration in terra incognita, is to invite people in all eras and from all faiths on an introspective adventure that is nothing less than an ontological transmutation, the fusion of humans into beings of excellence—the living ideal, *deva deha*—referred to in India's sacred writings.

2
Science and Spirituality

Mysticism is above all an experience that cannot be learned from books. A profound understanding of any mystical tradition can only be obtained when one decides to become actively involved in it.

Fritjof Capra, *The Tao of Physics*

For anyone who sees the Truth as a rich, unexplored country, the choice of pathway to attain it seems secondary. This is without doubt the explanation for the bifurcation during the Renaissance of a path that was common to the East and the West. While the East followed a centripetal way to enlightenment via the elimination of the sensory world through introspection, the West, with its technological discoveries enriched by the theories of the Age of Enlightenment, opted for a centrifugal expansionism designed to lead it to the same Truth, an approach that was in reality one of defiant deviance from past traditions, a kind of materialistic agnosticism.

No one could regret this separation, any more than one could lament a similar division that occurred at the dawn of Western history when we threw in our lot with Aristotle, the father of analytical knowledge and the realism of things, rather than with the other great sage of the time, Heraclitus of Ephesus, for whom the becoming of every being is made of nonbeing. This is the same Heraclitus, presented in Sri Aurobindo's monograph, and in Osho's book *The Hidden Harmony,* as a great mystic, who seemed to recognize the inextricable unity of the eternal and the transitory—"everything flows; nothing remains [still]"—that which is forever yet seems to exist only in this strife and change, which is a continuous dying.

The vocational "Whys" of science started probably with the basic cosmological question "Why is there something rather than nothing?" Granted that things *do* exist, the corollary question of "How?" inevitably emerges. Assuming an isomorphic confluence between the immensely vast cosmos and the animal kingdom at large, and more particularly human beings, we may next question if there is a possible correlation between today's prevailing theory of a constantly expanding universe and human evolution. At a more concrete level, we may also wish to plunge into the lesser-known aspects of sleep, a phenomenon shared by all living beings, and which in human life obliterates as much as one-third of our life span. Could this "unproductive" time, which corresponds to a state of nonexistence to the outer world, have a deeper cause and meaning than simply the recovery of biological and mental energies lost during the daytime?

Science, which functions today as a new order of planetary evangelist, most often subjected to utilitarian aspirations, has for a long time brandished the banner of "progress" in opposition to religious obscurantism. At the same time, it proposes an objective explanation of the reality of the world, subject nevertheless to increasingly burdensome investments and a profusion of tools for which the bar in innovation and performance never ceases to be raised. The illusory promise of science experienced a reversal due to the arrival of quantum theory with its lack of deterministic causality, which raises an insurmountable obstacle to objectivist techno-utopians.

We can obviously admit that, in spite of their differences, both the traditional approach and contemporary research ultimately intend to uncover the truth, the former in a union of the human and the Divine, the latter in the technical knowledge of manifestation. This simple postulate could be considered as a "positive synthesis" (along the lines of Hegel's proposal to reconcile thesis and antithesis into a synthesis).

Two Paths of Evolution

We must nevertheless remember the fundamental distinctions that separate these two paths. The doctrine of Yoga rests on an understanding of evolution that is the opposite of Darwin's theory. It considers itself holistic and aims at the future of the human, whose nature is hidden and divine. Physical science, on the other hand, as Max Planck said, progresses one funeral at a time. Its purpose is nothing more than a never ending litany of research going in all directions. It generally adheres to Darwinian theory by setting as its intention an experimental and speculative orientation, which is, by necessity, utilitarian.

At the level of methodology, we should especially note that the first of these paths is of an involuting nature, like a spiral movement going toward its center or origin. It refuses or minimizes the impact of materiality and does not depend on any instrumentation other than that of a mind dedicated to introspection, with a duty to avoid the subtle traps of mental projection in its final objective of attaining a state of genuine enlightenment. The ancient science of Yoga does not need any support (scientific or speculative) to explain, confirm, and justify the transcendence of its spirituality.

The second path is still largely linked to an evolutionary foundation, with its exclusive dependence on the intellect, reasoning, and myriad technologies. Its prevailing environment is determined by fierce competition and the attitude of world conqueror that comes from its Western heritage. Globalization opens the doors of the numerous riches of our technological civilization to all the inhabitants of the planet, without regard to social, racial, or other distinctions. It offers thousands of products and services that touch every area of modern life. And, like a child discovering his surroundings, the modern-day Ulysses knows the constant temptation to yield to the Sirens in an ocean of technical marvels whose polymorphous song never ceases.

However, the "truth" of our life constantly challenges logic, reason, and the numerous psychoanalytical methods in fashion in the past or present. The human tragedy resides as much in the fate of our ineluctable physical death as in the feeble means of personal investigation at our disposal, limited as they are to a four-dimensional relativistic continuum and a short life span. We are handicapped by our mental conditioning, modestly equipped with five senses of perception, and limited by an unreliable intuition. While apparatus and instruments for exploring the secrets of matter and the universe push back the limits indefinitely, they are often deployed at high cost and given top priority, despite the major challenges that we face with a suffering biosphere and the enduring social misery that surrounds us. Once we try to understand the true nature of the physical world that shelters us and the mind that we inhabit (and which dominates us), we discover that this approach leaves us at best dissatisfied and at worst powerless.

Although Western physics does not have the same objectives as the esoteric aspect of Yoga, there is no opposition between the two. There are even certain points of convergence and a common language—up to the point, however, of the mystical experience, which is rarely expressed in the ordinary or rational terms of the physical sciences. In these times of globalization, it even appears that the sciences are becoming mystical and researchers of mystical experience becoming more scientific.

In an interview with Renée Weber (titled "Physicist and Mystic—Is a Dialogue Between Them Possible?"), David Bohm, one of the most eminent theoretical physicists of our time, explained that "the positive meaning of mysticism is that the very foundation of our experience is a mystery—an assertion accepted by Einstein himself. He [Einstein] said mystery is the most beautiful thing. In my opinion, however, the term *mystic* should be applied only to whoever has a direct experience of the mystery that transcends the possibility of what can be described. For the rest of us it remains to be discovered what that means." Elsewhere he emphasized "the coherence that exists between the physicist and the mystic, the common view of an implicit order and an ocean of energy, which evolves into the creation of space, time, and matter."

In any event, scientific experimentation is insufficient to know anything other than the parts of the whole. On the other hand, the spiritual mystical experience tends toward a whole, integral understanding of everything. The first is founded on dialectical thought and analysis based on temporal patterns. The second, which claims to be holistic and whose *modus operandi* is apperception, is interested in an implicit dimension based on nontemporal universal principles.

The Possibility of Fusion

Given the current state of understanding, the fusion of these two fundamentally disparate methods seems hard to achieve. In a universe where we are the hostages of relativity, one could note the fact that, in spite of the current wave of globalization and the forms of rapid communication that accompany it, the level of knowledge on our planet still remains very mixed. Human advances, whether materialistic or spiritual, are never general and homogenous. Progress often varies widely, not only at the individual level, but also in terms of societies or civilizations. Levels of awareness concerning the realities of the world and life values differ in a significant manner. So it is in this pluralistic world of biodiversity, dominated by a materialistic search for happiness, that at the same instant a man lands on the moon, other men in Australia and the Amazon still live in the Stone Age, in total ignorance of the buzz of the technologically oriented world surrounding them. Therefore, is it unreasonable to imagine certain evolved humans on the verge of having an experience that is diametrically opposed to that of the surrounding world, and yet not ignoring it? Sri Aurobindo is said to have claimed that the yogi is a being whose consciousness is situated several thousand years ahead of contemporary humanity.

History teaches that Alexander the Great was the inventor of the term *Hindu,* which is the origin of the name *India* today. During one of his expeditions this young disciple of Aristotle discovered the "gymnosophists," naked ascetics, Hindu ancestors of the elite yogic ascetics today known as *naga nagas* or *naga babas*. Since this period of antiquity, Yoga has always been considered the chosen ground of the *siddhis,* these extraordinary realizations that defy numerous physical and psychological laws and that always surprise us despite rational research into the question. How can we explain yogic phenomenology at a time of modern technological prowess and the communication that accompanies it?

The fundamental purpose of the *āsanas* is to establish a motionless and comfortable attitude for mental concentration. With grace, control, and purity, the following pictures highlight typical *āsanas* in standing, prone, inverted, and sitting postures.

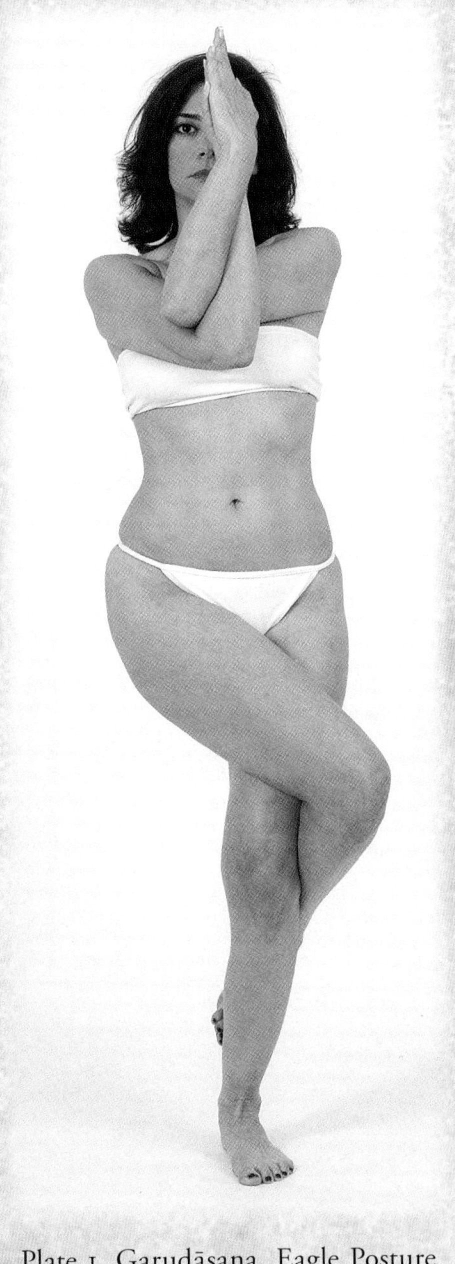

Plate 1. Garuḍāsana, Eagle Posture

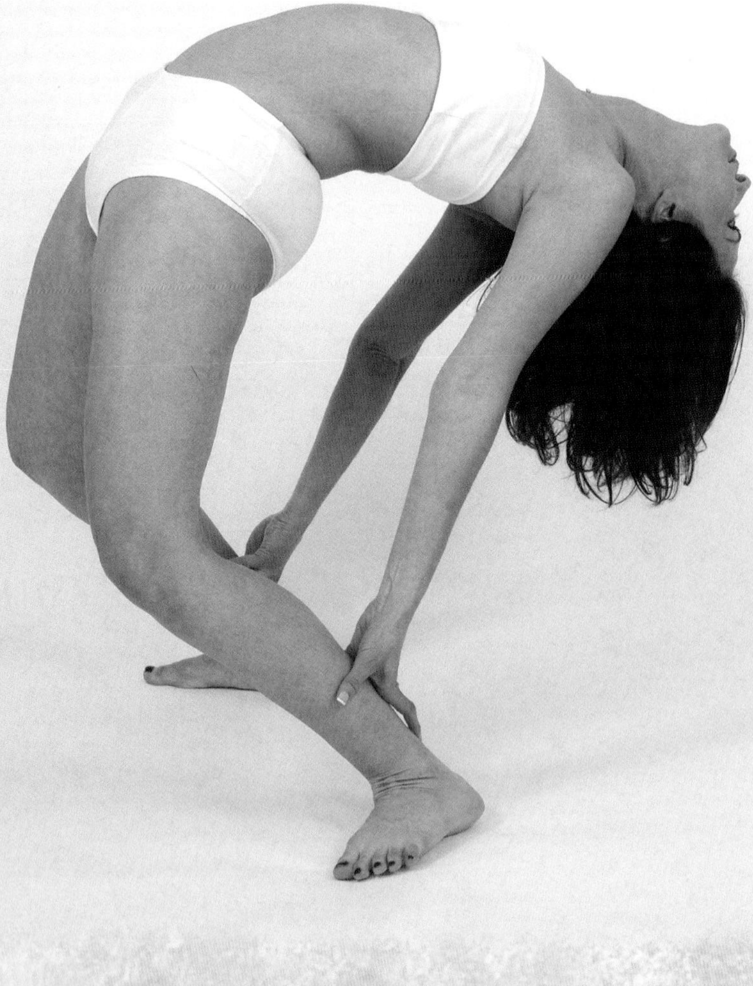

Plate 2. Pṛiṣṭhāsana, Back Posture

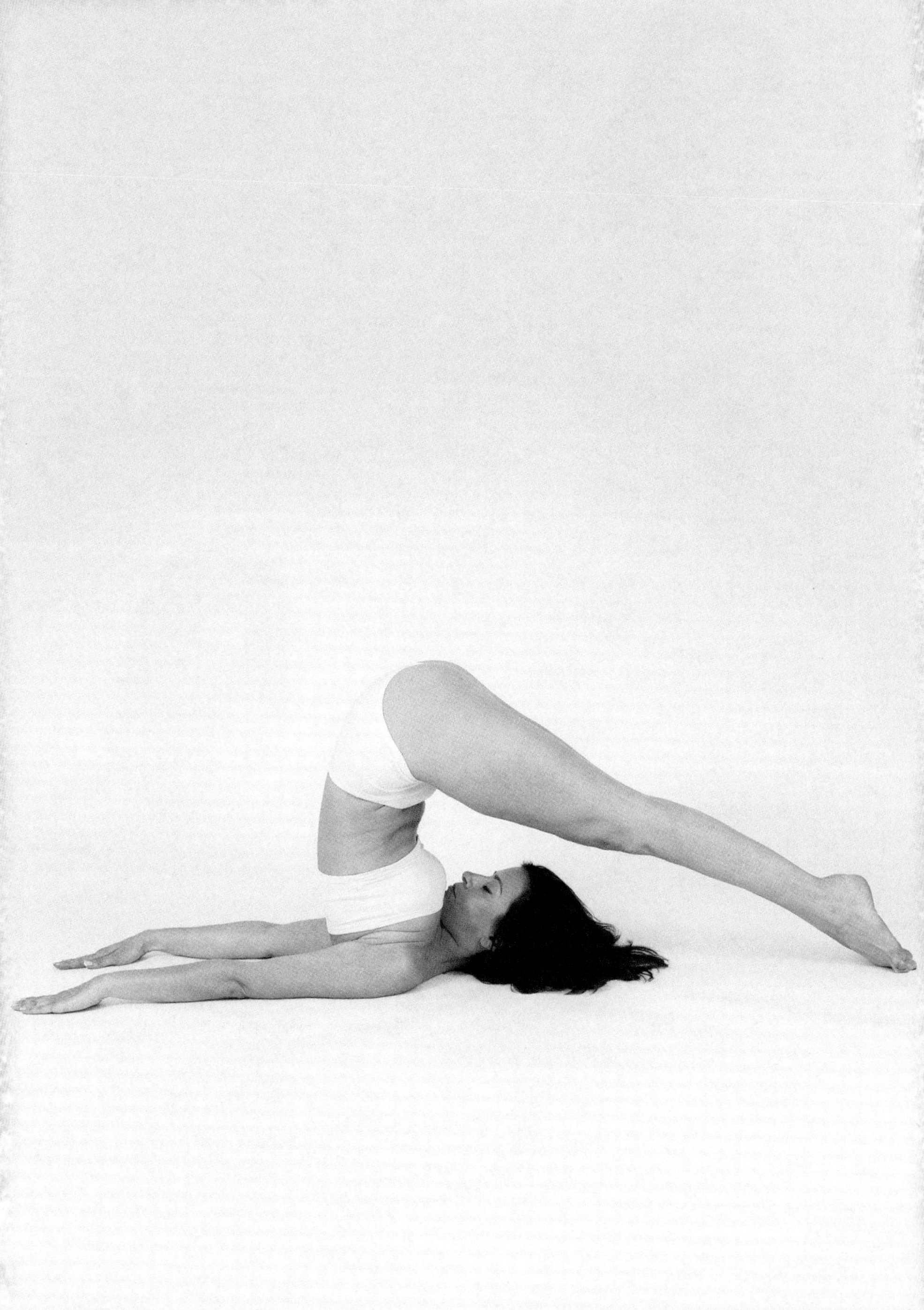

Plate 3. Halāsana, Plow Posture

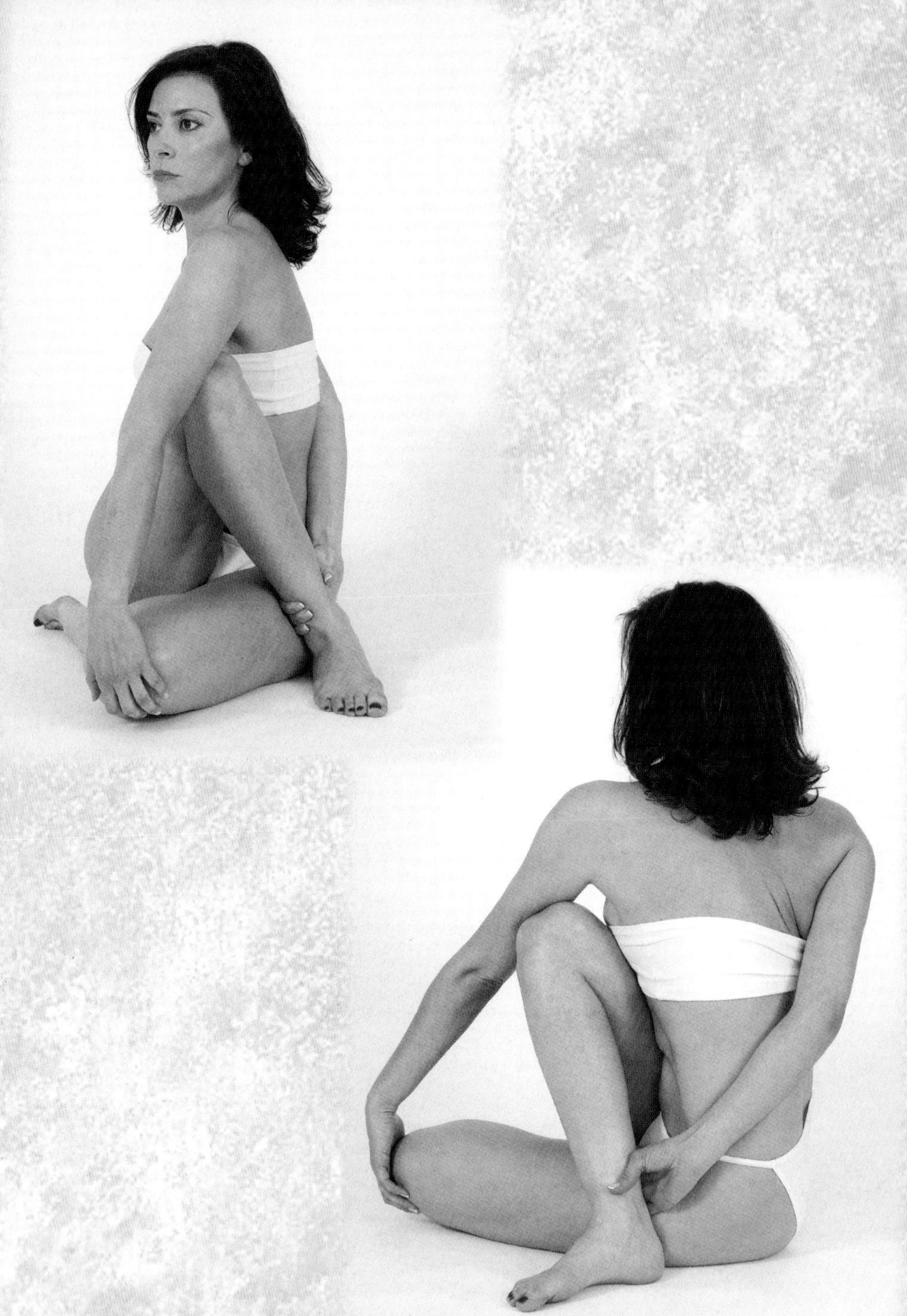

Plate 4. Baddha Ardha Matsyendrāsana,
Ankle-Hold Modified Spinal-Twist Posture

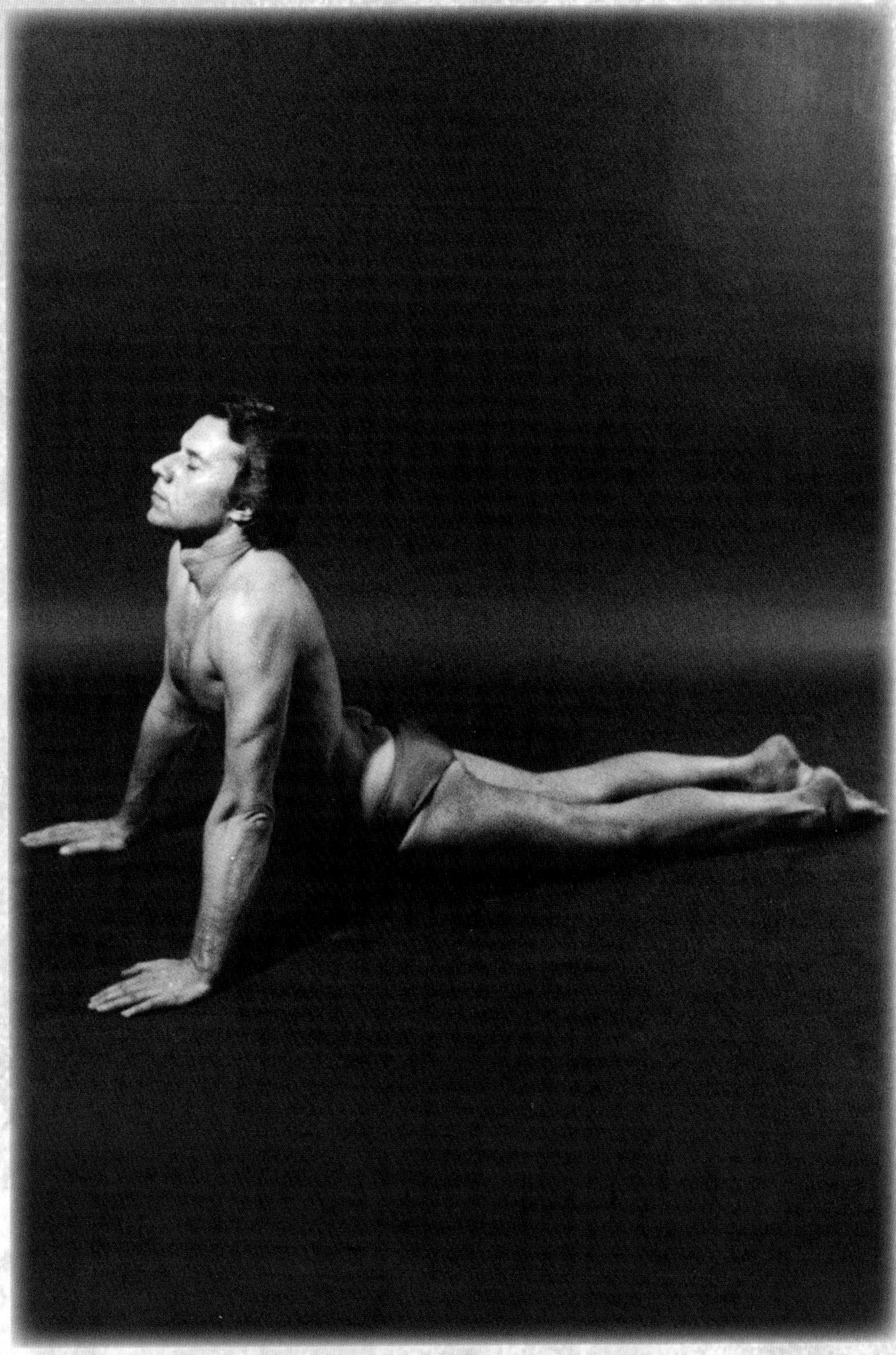

Plate 5. Bhujangāsana, Cobra Posture

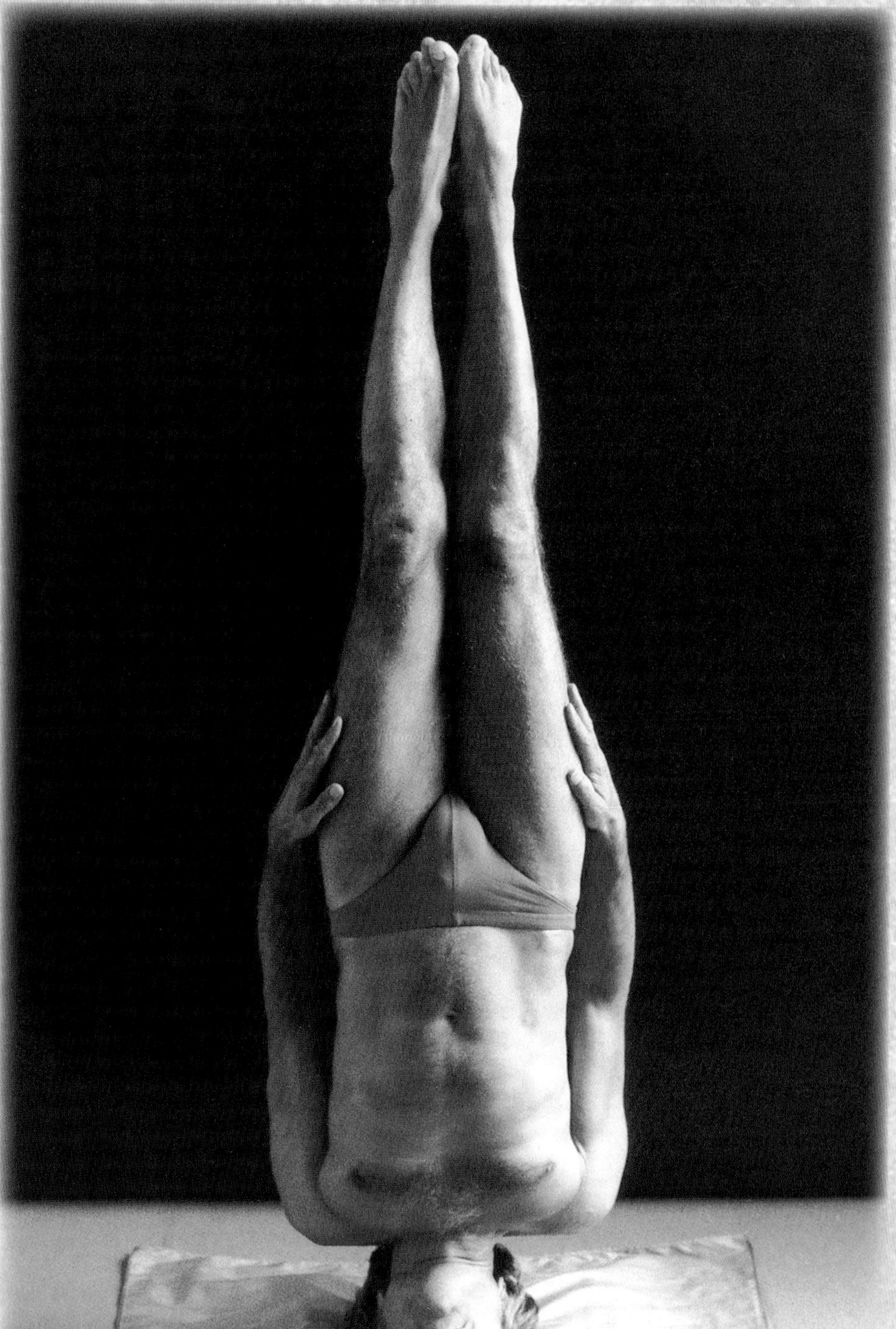

Plate 6. Śirāsana, Head-Stand Posture

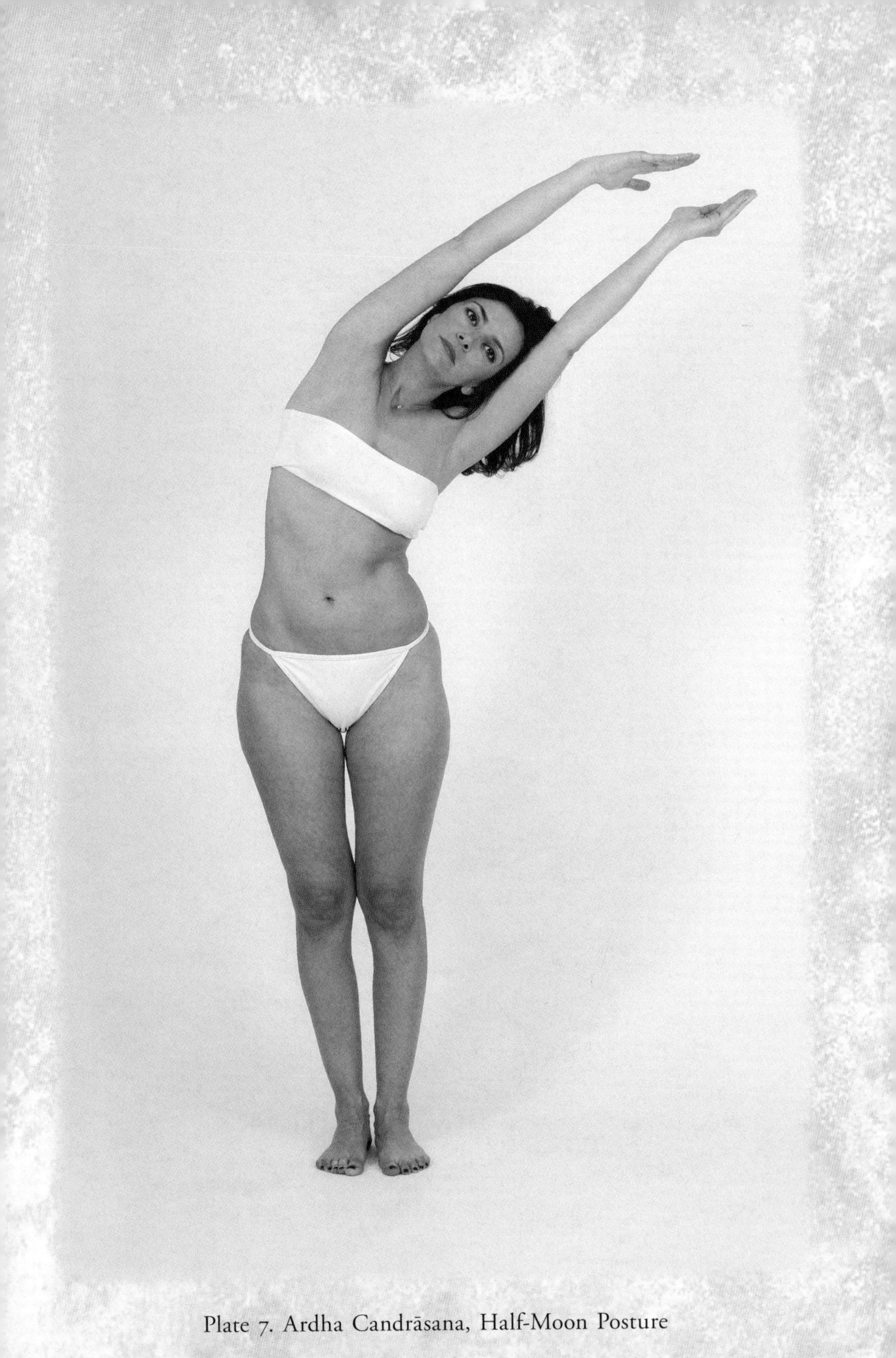

Plate 7. Ardha Candrāsana, Half-Moon Posture

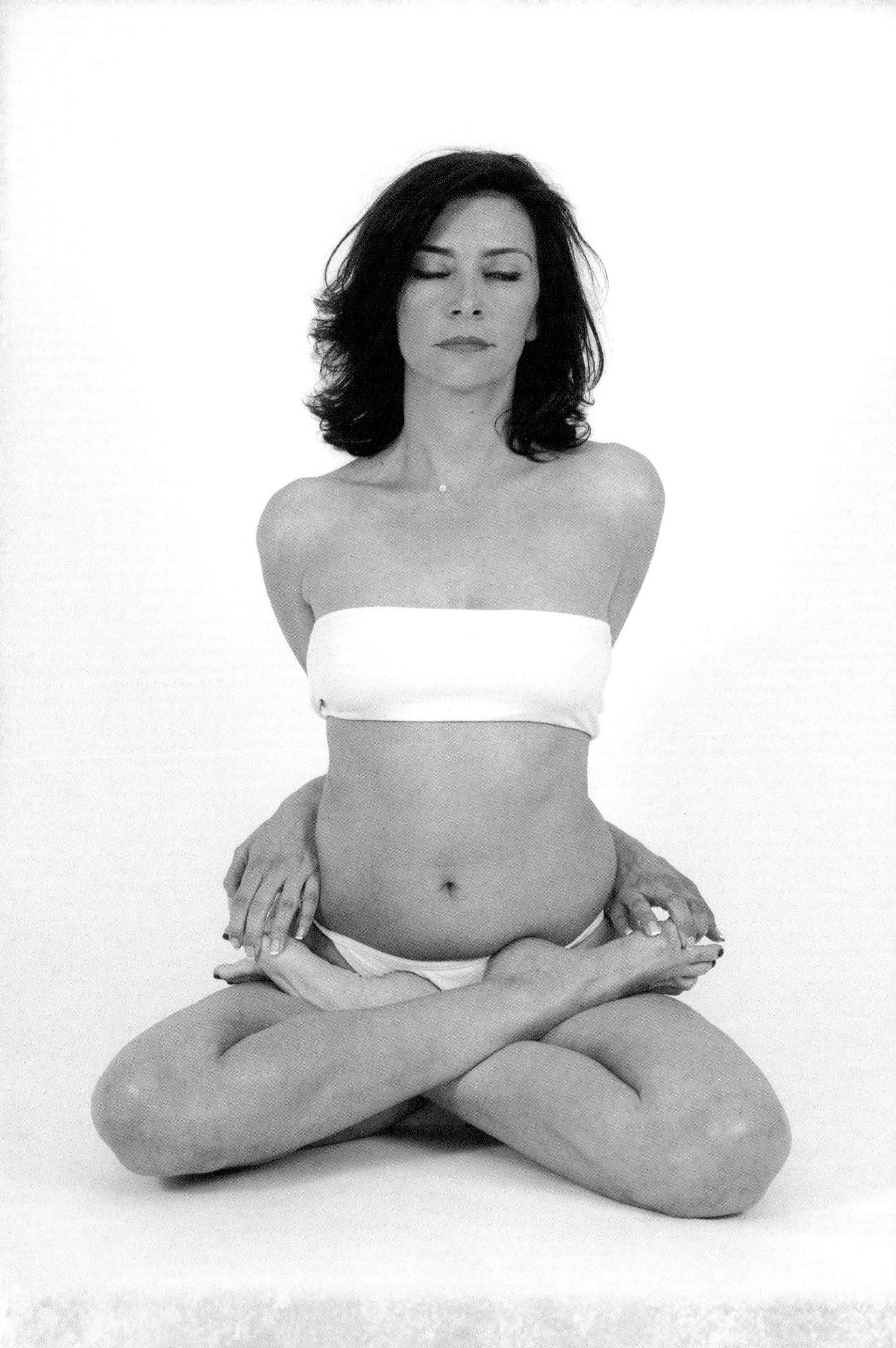

Plate 8. Baddha Padmāsana, Toe-Hold Lotus Posture

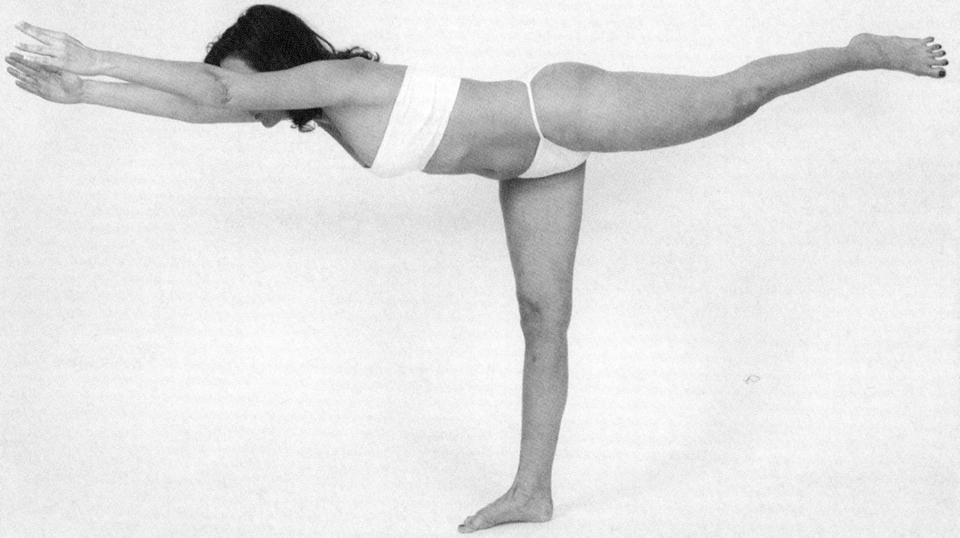

Plate 9. Ekapādāsana, Single-Foot Posture

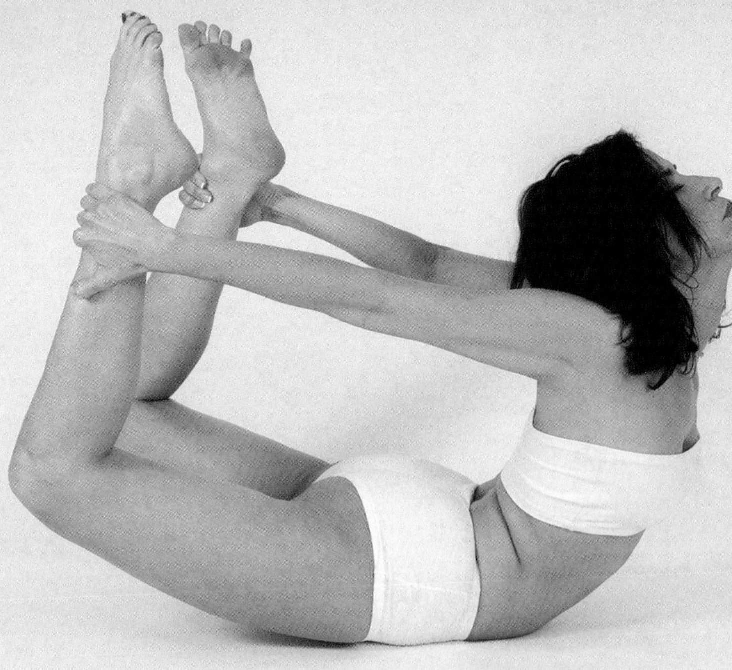

Plate 10. Dhanurāsana, Bow Posture

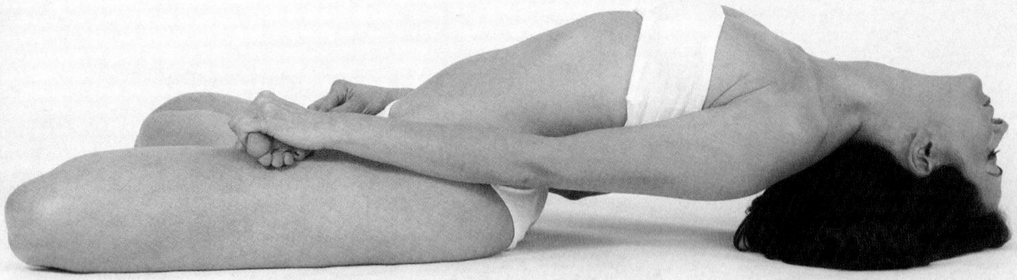

Plate 11. Matsyāsana, Fish Posture

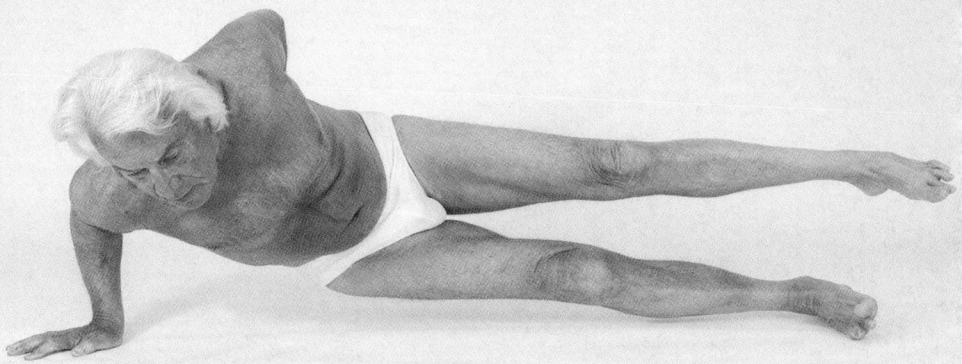

Plate 12. Bāhu-pādāsana, (or Dvipādāsana), Arm-Leg Posture

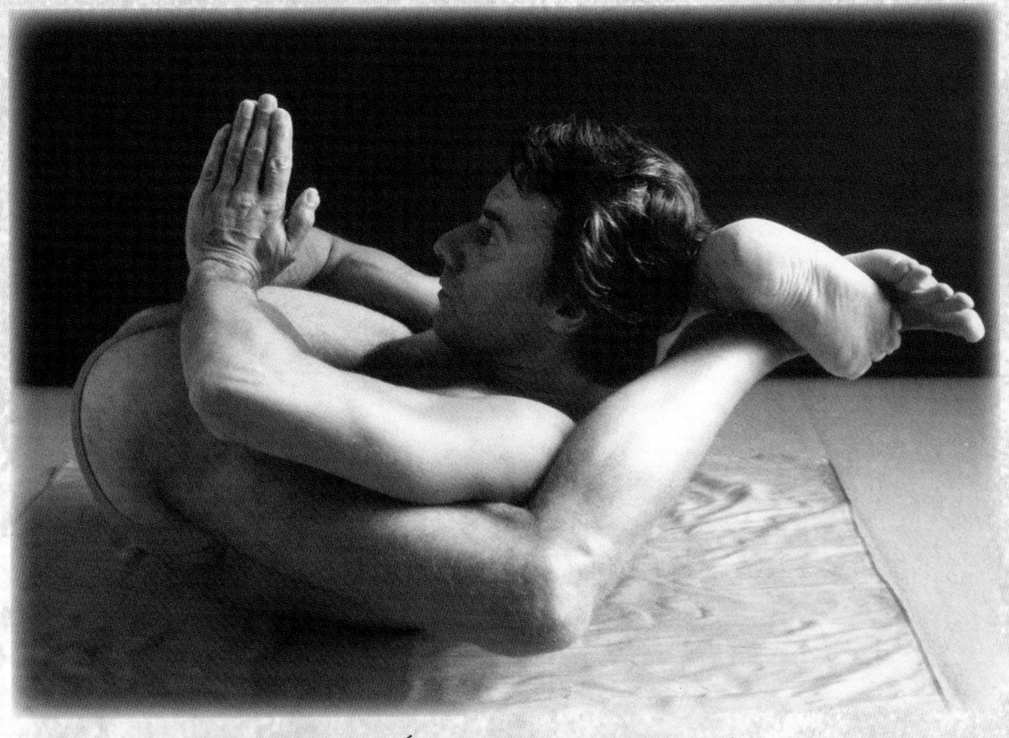

Plate 13. Dvipāda Śirāsana, Double Foot-Head Posture

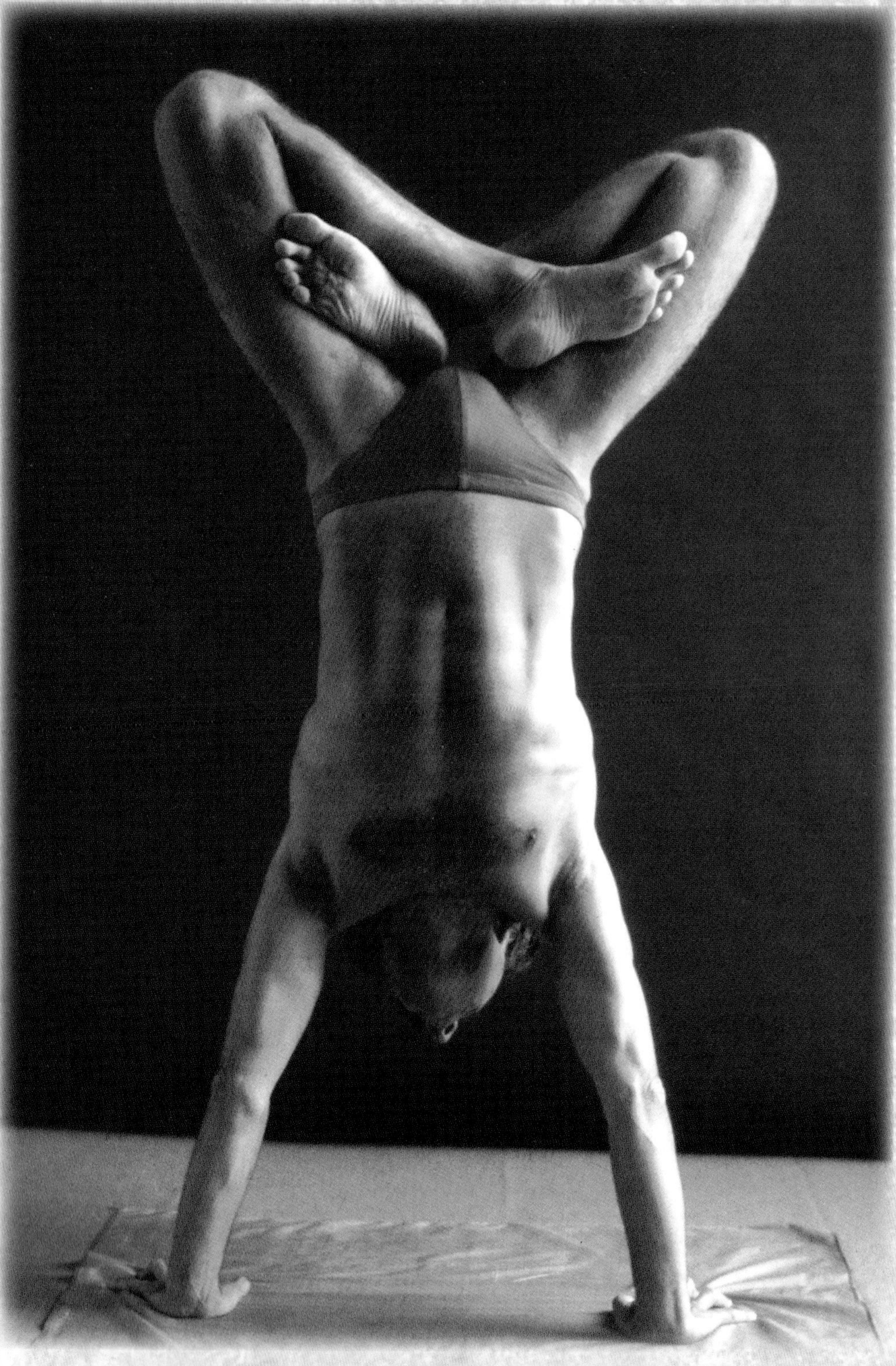

Plate 14. Hastapadma Vṛiksāsana, Arm-Stand Lotus Posture

In India the yogi(ni) starts the day with a morning prayer and dedicates all forthcoming thoughts and actions to the Divine. The yogi(ni) cultivates a most cherished *deva deha* ideal by offering all efforts, mental and physical, on the altar of his or her *sādhana*. Traditional Haṭha Yoga training commences with a silent confirmation of the morning prayer. The gentle spiritual warrior bows head thankfully to the beloved guru whose know-how, heritage, and presence, living or posthumous, are a continuous source of inspiration.

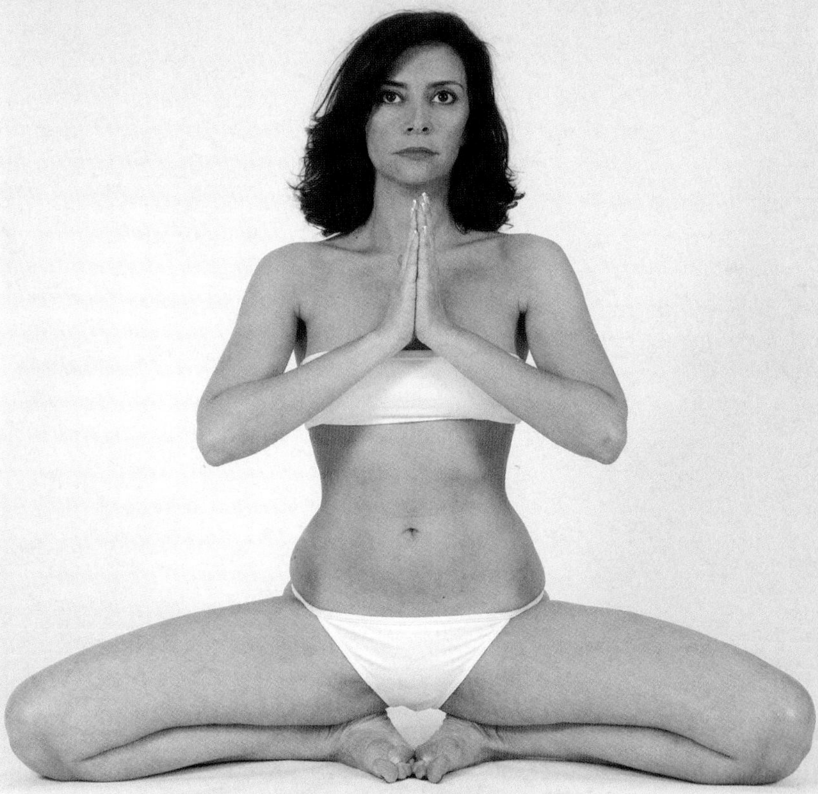

Plate 15. Bhadrāsana, Happy Posture

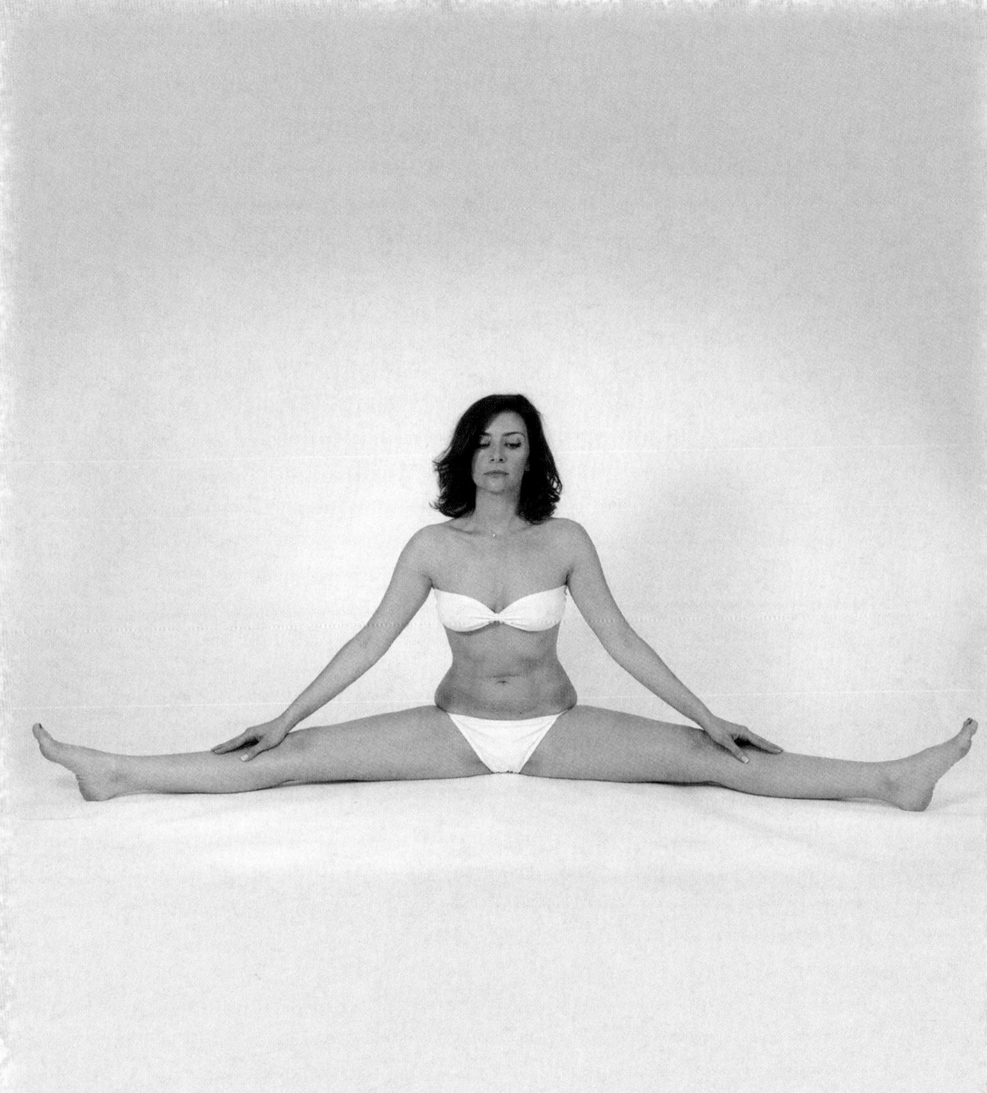

Plate 16. Pādaprasāraṇāsana, Sideward Leg-Stretch Posture

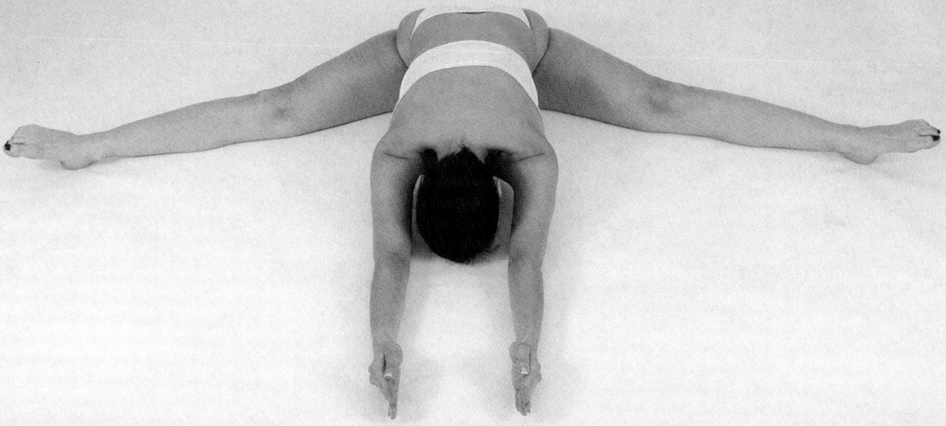

Plate 17. Praṇatāsana, Forward Body-Bend Posture

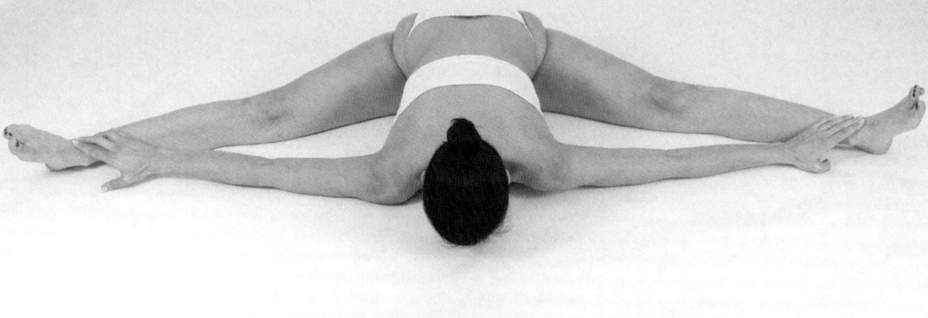

Plate 18. Nataśirāsana, Head-Bend Posture

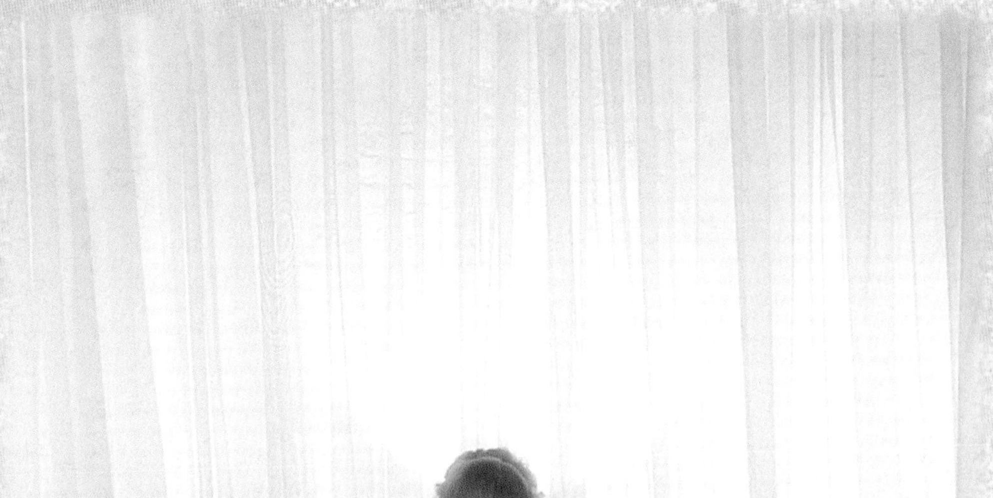

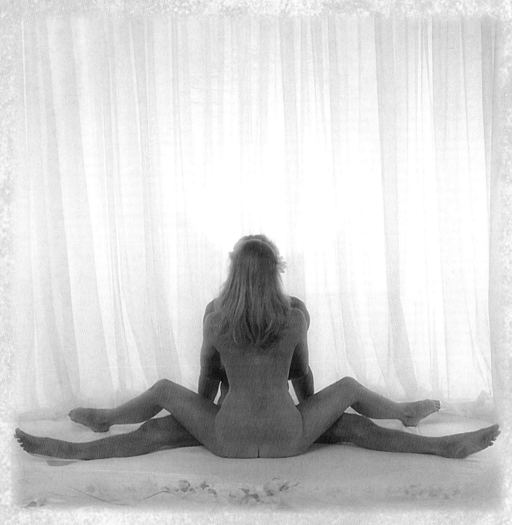

Plate 19. Maithuna, the sacred act, which allows an all-absorbing union with the beloved one, the *devatā*.

A concern for objectivity invites suggestion rather than prognostication based on scattered observations and some experienced Indians' confidentially entrusted secrets. It seems, however, that these issues should be approached with other considerations in mind:

1. The incompatible nature of diametrically opposed research programs gives rise to a lack of agreement between the self-proclaimed scientific objectivity of the Western researcher and the transcendence of the tangible world that is proclaimed by the yogi.
2. The absence of reference points and criteria of methodological evaluation.
3. The empirical limitations of a medico-scientific methodology whose aim is essentially to observe abnormal or pathological behaviors as opposed to the "supranormality" of the yogi.
4. The small population of candidates possessing *siddhis* does not constitute a scientifically valid test sample.
5. The yogi's obvious lack of interest in being submitted to tests that are not designed to help him progress in his *sādhana* or, in his view, to improve human health.

In addition, yogis are sometimes aware of the experimental criteria used in scientific research, which is often split by competition or is the victim of trends and pressures. Another important barrier, this time to do with cultural history, is the regrettable and notorious arrogance of certain scientists who are infatuated with their academic merits, the fact that they live in a rich country, and, in the worst cases, the belief that they belong to a superior race. Nevertheless, the extraordinary feats of the *siddhis* surprise us with the mastery and psychic force that is involved.

Why should we thus be surprised at the difficulty of resolving a relationship that, instead of allowing an enriching complementarity, revives the question of the dialogue between the two historically antagonistic, epistemological styles of West and East, tangible and intangible, materialism and spirituality. Rather than lingering vainly on the "miraculous" character of unexplained *siddhis,* the honest researcher will undoubtedly prefer to be astonished at the age-old capacity for survival of an essentially oral tradition in an impermanent world, a tradition without any institutional structure, which has been able to surmount the vicissitudes of earthly temporal, political, and religious power.

In fact, the present-day dualism between modern scientific or religious thought, on the one hand, and the Hindu tradition, on the other, illustrates the axiom according to which two parallel lines can never intersect. Undeniably, all attempts to bring harmony between cultures or religions are highly laudable, as is mutual tolerance, social justice, or the vision of people enjoying peaceful coexistence. Any effort at rapprochement therefore deserves encouragement so as to develop real solidarity and provide a link allowing the elimination of North-South barriers and filling the ancient chasm that for several centuries has separated the East from the West.

3
Yoga in Daily Life

A Lack of Mastery

Our daily life unfolds in a scattered mental world. Our mind, this marvelous feature of our inner world, the most important one in our lives, is incapable of concentrating or relaxing. It incessantly seeks objects, goals, chimera . . . Sometimes we are repulsed by the inability of our mind to remain still, but our powerlessness, our weakness, makes us incapable of mastering our continual mental movement.

Even when we satisfy our existential needs for food and lodging, we nevertheless remain dissatisfied. Moreover, to satisfy our needs, whether they are genuine or not, we are too often ready to indulge in great excesses. We seem to have no capacity for adapting to what we truly need. We have quite simply allowed our excesses to shape our environment to the point where it influences the whole of our mental life.

Most of our thoughts are never expressed, for we do not have the strength to give them form and allow them to bear fruit. As a result, many of these thoughts will have an effect that is opposite to the one intended; and yet, we cannot prevent ourselves from thinking them. Why is that? This inability is expressed in low self-confidence, a feeling of uncertainty, and lack of spiritual courage. It is revealed in all our indulgences, our limitations, our narrow viewpoints, and our unfulfilled desires. And that is not all. Our body cannot tolerate indefinitely these material excesses. At a certain point, a process of physical destruction commences. The nervous system can no longer resist the irritations to which it is subjected. The body loses its vitality, weakens, and becomes sickly.

We have absolutely no chance of resisting the huge pressure of our thoughts, actions, emotional reactions, worries, and failures. We lack enough strength to deal with the challenges of our lifestyle. We tremble and withdraw when confronted with the prospect of having to swim across an ocean of activities. We stagger under the responsibility of a difficult job and we collapse when the results are not what were expected. If the reverses in life do not strengthen our courage, harden us, and make us even more determined, it is a sign that we need to renew the strength of our spiritual resistance.

We forget the misuse to which we subject our body and mind in our daily life, the fact that certain forces are liberated, whereas others, though related, are left unused. This means that we have lost control of our "direction." One part of our energy is therefore poorly utilized. All this results in a scattered mind, wrapped up in logic, which leads to an ongoing dissipation of our inner force. We have only to consider the situations in which we are dominated by a strong emotion, incapable of controlling it; this is a sign that we lack the necessary mastery, that our disjointed mind never ceases to waste its energy.

To live solely on the material plane, without taking into account mental and spiritual values, is to risk a regrettable debasement of the self. If the acquisition of muscular strength and the health of internal organs are not accompanied by clear thinking and a balanced emotional life, an insidious fall inevitably awaits us. When the spiritual brake is not in operation, we are seriously affected by dietary, sexual, and other excesses.

Accessing the Infinite According to Yoga

To oppose the destructive effect of such imbalance and to protect ourselves physically, morally, and spiritually, we need Yoga in our daily life. The inner being, seat of enormous forces, is highly stimulated by Yoga. We must plumb the depths of our existence and find the laws that, even if inactive, are nevertheless crucial in the limited framework of what we can understand and grasp in our daily life. It is there that we find true strength. Moreover, this force must be tempered in an optimal manner through the practice of Yoga.

To begin at the very beginning, we must first accept the present condition of our mind and body. Our goal is to control the central internal force that, in the end, puts us in a position to access the infinite essence of peace and eternal bliss. To attain such a goal, intensive training of our concentration is necessary in order to give birth, via the awakening of forces that sleep within us, to a purified body endowed with the greatest vitality. On a level beyond the sensory, certain signs then appear, which penetrate the knowable world and the infinity beyond. Yoga is a method that has been systematically tested for this noble goal.

Life then appears more beautiful, refined, and rich. It becomes the source of happiness, and the mind also becomes more clear, tranquil, peaceful, and emotionally satisfied. If its precepts are followed with intelligence and regularity, the discipline of Yoga brings to the body cleanliness, freshness, vitality, and strength.

Physical Conditions of the Spiritual Life

> *No amount of sermonizing or sophistication, of intellectuality or intuition, subtlety or simplicity, free thinking or determinism, will ever bring you a step nearer the accomplishment of your object, if that is the attainment of peace of mind, so long as there is disease in your body.*
>
> Jatindra Mohana
> (Sri S. S. Goswami's father)

Experience teaches us that a body whose hygiene is neglected, whose health vacillates, and which suffers from weakness or lack of mastery cannot become the support of a superior mental life nor withstand the constraints of daily life. Our mental and spiritual life is inseparably linked to our physical life. Of course, it is possible to acquire a certain amount of strength and functional effectiveness of both the autonomous nervous system and the muscular system without a corresponding development of the mental and spiritual aspects, but it is then only a superficial achievement. Such a state corresponds to a human life that regresses toward that of primates, which is a form of evolution lacking survival value—in effect, a sort of biological degradation.

In reality, human mental and spiritual development has great biological value specific to our species. In Yoga, this individual twofold aim transcends Karl Marx's affirmation: "The free development of each is the condition for the free development of all." Yoga affords the possibility of bringing forth human beings who are flourishing fully and harmoniously. In Haṭha Yoga the aim sought is, more specifically, to develop a physical body that is ideally adapted to mental concentration and to a superior life of the mind, while conserving optimal functionality and effectiveness. This physical form favors above all a healthy body. Health does not consist solely in avoiding illness, as important as that may seem. Good health is a state in which all the organs function flawlessly in a harmonious symbiosis.

Yogic Sublimity

The human body is a genuine marvel, but its true destiny is not on the physical level. Even if human beings managed to develop their bodies to the impressive dimensions of mythological giants, the body would not be their real grandeur. Trying to evaluate humans uniquely in terms of physical achievements makes no sense. Our true nature cannot be attained in this way.

Our real essence resides in our mind, a world in itself that we constantly renew and which gives us the possibility of growing well beyond our supposed limits. It is this creative force that is unique to human beings. The very survival of the human species depends on it. Our grandeur or banality, our constitution or anatomy, our broad- or narrow-mindedness, our perspicacity or blindness, our desires and tendencies, our representations of the world and our ideas, in fact everything of which we are composed, is determined by our aspirations, thinking, and feelings. It is the specific character of our thoughts that defines our mental life and our entire nature. Human beings are completely reflected in their own thoughts.

In daily life, thoughts generally lead to survival or circumstantial objectives of questionable nature. Often greed, envy, boasting, vanity, frivolity, lust, debauchery, hyperactivity, and self-deception constitute the mental life. People at this stage express an inferior level of thought. Their emotional life is out of control, their morality remains undeveloped, and their spirituality lies fallow, so to speak. Such individuals are chained by their narrow conception of life, which features other negative properties such as egotism, illness, worry, and a lack of self-assurance, linked to the fear of failure, which causes health hazards with great physical and mental suffering. We can clearly discern in this suffering the pernicious effects of an unsatisfactory lifestyle. Moreover, such misfortunes are only part of the painful price that people like this will have to pay. Yoga describes this stage as one of hyperactivity and sensory blindness.

However, there are more elevated stages in which a person's thoughts are more constructive and stronger, although most often the activities of such individuals are very much one-sided. For example, there are people who, having developed great physical strength, have success in athletics and sports, or else individuals who, having attained a particularly elevated mental maturity, evolve effortlessly in the world of ideas. Those who hold physical beauty and strength as an ideal have effectively proven that the human body possesses considerable latent capacities. However, unable to appreciate the value of developing in a harmonious fashion, they pay heavy tribute to their high-level specialty. There are also people who have remarkable lucidity and a fertile imagination, whether as artists, scientists, businessmen, or geniuses. Nevertheless, even they are not always in harmony because, though they have reached the heights of the mental life, they have neglected other aspects, such as the body.

On the other hand, there are individuals with elevated aspirations who live in another mental world. They do not judge things with the yardstick of materialistic criteria, and they do not give themselves the goal of earthly success. They are not satisfied with the joys to which we aspire, and they are not affected by the reverses, suffering, and worries from which we try to flee. They are not concerned with riches or material goods, to which others devote their lives. Poverty and other difficulties, which subjugate and crush most of us, do not frighten them. From these purified and beautiful beings who radiate spiritual light, a call often emerges to transcend the dualistic conditions of human life and chart the path of Self-realization.

Once we are really aware of the possibility of reaching such a different state of mind, and at the moment we are prepared to meet the ever-challenging yogic admonition "Know Thyself," preferably under the guidance of a competent and experienced Yoga teacher, we should not hesitate to give ourselves a good start. For most of us, the yogic path chosen will not imply a monastic life, and there is no need to give up the social dimensions of modern life such as family, career, community obligations, and so on. Many advanced yogis have reached high spiritual goals as Middle Way seekers, that is, by being fully involved in both the profane area and the sacred path of *sādhana*.

However, to elude possible conflicts and a strenuous progression, it may be wise to inform those to whom we are intimately committed about our decision to live a twofold life, something that may not always be understood by those who are satisfied with an incidental lifestyle. Also, it is indispensable to find a harmonious *modus vivendi* by adopting a smart plan that fairly partitions the time and energy that is dedicated to social life and to spiritual search.

At the intellectual level, it is essential to once and for all accept that purity is a must and, from the outset, to discard lingering flummery and futile illusions, lest we soon be deluded about the results expected. Yoga *sādhana* should not be undertaken with a view to acquiring extraordinary human powers.

Serious seekers of Truth in the yogic tradition start their spiritual journey by accepting certain basic prerequisites such as faith and belief in the theory of rebirth, which are a necessary ideological frame in addition to full confidence in one's spiritual guide. The great adventure of Yoga *sādhana* supposes sustained efforts without anticipating results according to a particular time frame. This does not mean that tangible results may not be experienced at an early stage of the practice.

A Middle East erudite once attended a lecture on Yoga I gave in his country. To his query on the benefits one may expect from Yoga *sādhana,* I replied:

> Have you ever experienced a different reveille, waking up as if from a prolonged sweet dream, or the aftermath of a harmonious union, bathing in the unexplainable feeling of untinged happiness ?
>
> Have you ever had, all of sudden, a genial insight, delving into unfathomable depths, or attained the peaks of elevated thoughts, in loneliness?
>
> Have you ever experienced the spontaneous feeling of an elevated harmony beyond words, associated with strength and mastery?
>
> Have you ever been immersed in the emotion of an all-pervading and seemingly timeless love toward no one in particular and toward everyone, alive or dead, human or animal, plants and trees, toward the whole universe?

Do you say "Yes"? Surely you are one of the privileged hearts, yogis and sages who in all ages, from time immemorial, have attained desirable heights in the search for the Self.

If you say "No," don't be sorry, but don't waste time. Follow the wise Upaniṣadic advice "Arise, seek a teacher, and endeavor to know who you are."

4
Yama–Ethical Rules

The ten ethical rules of *yama* and *niyama* constitute the foundation and moral basis for every serious aspirant (or accomplished yogi) whose ambitions aim higher than the benefits of health and well-being (which are easily acquired with this discipline). For certain people, they also restrain the ambition to attain the superhuman powers that yogis sometimes experience. A superior Yoga practice supposes a superior personal moral order; all the same, this morality is not necessarily comparable to civic or religious morality. In a spirit of mastery, accompanied by the blessing of a spiritual master, yogis and yoginis submit to strict rules that enable them to lift the veil of illusion and ignorance inherent in human nature.

The Vedic origin of the term *yama* is affirmed in the Samhītās and Brāhmaṇas, and most particularly in the famous Yoga aphorisms of Patañjali (II.30–32). *Yama* covers five rules directed toward others, in other words, rules that regulate social behavior: *ahimsā* (abstinence from injury), *satya* (truthfulness), *asteya* (abstinence from theft), *brahmacarya* (sexual control in thought, emotion, and action), and *aparigraha* (noncovetousness).

Ahimsā

This first rule requires refraining from all physical, verbal, or mental violence. There is evidently no universal code of conduct that permits us to uniformly adjust our behavior to the thousands of situations in daily life. A glass of water can save a life in one case and turn lethal in another. Depending on the place, time, and circumstances, what appears just in one context is no longer just in another. Each situation also reflects the person who is involved in it; it is unique and thus requires a lucid, measured approach based on reason or intuition.

The basis of Indian morality, *ahimsā* became a world-renowned movement thanks to Mahatma Gandhi who was able to apply it (along with the two next rules, *satya* and *asteya*) methodically and coherently, and achieve the hoped-for success in his struggle for the independence of his country. A pillar also of Buddhism and Jainism, the passive weapon of *ahimsā* has become an effective means of combat that has been adopted to this day by various ideological or political movements.

Satya

To be truthful is to be in strict alignment with what we perceive and think; it is to stick to the truth such as we experience it in the sensory or mental world. It distinguishes those persons, rare indeed, who are "integrated" beings. But there are certain particular situations where the observance of this rule is not easy. Thus taught Gautama Buddha, "You must never lie—unless you are a merchant," or unless this rule violates the preceding one of *ahimsā,* which consists in avoiding harm to others. To report faithfully an observed fact or an experienced situation is also part of this rule; it is violated if the report is deliberately modified or false.

Asteya

This rule, which in particular regulates the instinct of possessiveness and greed, facilitates the development of honesty. It consists of not stealing or appropriating in an illicit or immoral manner the possessions of others—physical or intangible.

Brahmacarya

This rule is undoubtedly the most important and also the most difficult of the ten ethical rules of *yama* and *niyama.* It is intimately related to that of *tapas,* whose multiple applications it oversees. The term *brahmacarya* appears notably in the *Bhāgavata,* the *Mahābhārata,* the *Rāmāyana,* and the *Yogavasiṣṭa.* It is also found in the *Yoga Sūtras* of Patañjali, the classic work of contemporary Yoga. Quoted no less than 177 times in the Yoga literature updated by Sri Shyam Sundar Goswami, this term appears frequently in the Purāṇas, where it designates the foundation of *sanātana dharma,* the eternal religion according to the *Brahmānanda Purāṇa* (63.31). This discipline is also referred to as "great wish" (*Skanda Purāṇa,* 6.237.12–15).

The discipline of *brahmacarya* is found in one form or another in all those who aspire to an elevated spiritual life and often in those who have gone through exceptional physical ordeals. Sri S. S. Goswami taught that *brahmacarya* is a method of total or partial sexual control, the aim of which is to preserve the vital force. In its aims and results, it clearly demonstrates the influence of the mind over the body.

In general, the process of procreation is intimately linked both to the pleasure obtained from sexual union and the prospect of seeing a child born. These two sources of pleasure constitute a natural human phenomenon. We cannot reasonably judge sexual union as an ugly, shameful act or, on the contrary, as a spiritual ideal in itself. It is possible to assert that sexual continence fails to serve the goal of Nature, namely the perpetuation of the species, and is therefore the opposite of a "normal" physical life; nevertheless, the fact remains that the voluntary cessation of the dissipation of sexual energy is justified in a spiritual quest. From the yogic point of view, it is considered of great value for the maintenance of a superior mental life.

The preservation of one's energy capital by sexual abstinence is found in all authentic expressions of spirituality. This preservation of the subtle human energy is in no way harmful, contrary to what is claimed by those who have usually never practiced it or who have made their observations only on sick subjects or those obsessed with sex. For cultural or medical reasons, sexual continence is seldom given an honorable place in modern societies, with the exception, however, of high level sports in which a practice of this kind is advocated.* In Asian and African traditions, in fact, this sacrifice is widely accepted once its objective pertains to high level sport.

In ancient and modern India, the experience of the advantages of abstinence, as taught by the rishis and yogis, is reinforced by the observation of the practitioners of *brahmacarya*. The yogic tradition, whose roots are in Āyurveda, the most ancient system of medicine in the world, emphasizes the importance of the *ojas*. Contrary to modern medicine, which (when it is not pretending to be unaware of it) identifies *ojas* as albumin or glucose, ancient Indian writings refer to it as a source of multiple benefits, notably for the brain and muscles. On the other hand, experience teaches that its dissipation is not without harmful effects: deterioration of organs, general weakness, decline of the sensory faculty, difficulty in mastering thoughts, anxiety, and bad health.

This ancient tradition considers the entire complexity of seminal energy, rather than simply focusing, as is the case today, on a substance of chemical composition that is especially rich in protein, fats, iron, and copper. It certainly has never viewed the fluid as some kind of detritus that the body is required to eject in order to remain in good health. Though the accumulation of organic wastes in the body turns out to be harmful to the organism, nothing on the other hand proves that the accumulation of sperm can be harmful. Abstinence is not the principal cause of a strong demand for the ejaculation of sperm. The seminal pressure starts in adolescence with the production of hormones, which continues up to a more or less advanced age in adults. Continence only brings this pressure into awareness. It is impossible to stop it.

Is it therefore abnormal to wish to master the flow of vital fluid

*For example, the U.S. World Boxing Champion "Sugar" Ray Robinson used to refrain from all sexual activity during a six-month period prior to major contests.

that plays both the biological role permitting procreation and the role of satisfying the need for sexual pleasure? And what can be said about the prolonged excessive loss of semen that clearly leads to the weakening of the body, often associated with a feeling of disgust and with sexual impotence, or which can be the cause of deficiency in the immune system in newborns?

In seminal energy, Yoga has discovered the primary aspect of its procreative function, *retas,* as well as a latent aspect, which, in the absence of any voluntary ejaculation, is stored in the genitals. In this last case, the vital substance called *ojas* appears in the yogi's body. In effect, thanks to the technique of *bindu-mārana,* which permits the contraction of the smooth muscle at the time of a strong accumulation of sperm, *retas* transforms into *ojas.* The conversion of *retas* into *ojas* using antiperistaltic movements (*urdhva-retas*) safeguards the energy dissipated in the sex act, effectively allowing the transmutation of substance into physical energy. The term *urdhva-retas* is frequently used to indicate the accomplished practitioner of this difficult discipline, which does not necessarily require strict celibacy.

It is perhaps fitting to mention here the popular materialistic idea formulated in the West that considers the Hindu *lingam* as a phallic symbol, whereas in fact it is primarily a symbolic representation of the conversion of sexual energy into life-force energy. Many physiological aspects deserve to be mentioned concerning the energetic conversion of *retas* into *ojas,* were it not for the limited scope of this brief presentation of *brahmacarya.*

It is important to remember that the sexual mastery involved in abstinence is measured on two levels: on the mental level, by a sincere motivation supported by an exceptional will, and on the physiological level. These two factors are synergistic: individual differences can be developed first of all on the mental level, when the adept manages to draw on different inspirational sources (spiritual guides, holy texts, or kinship with a group), as well as on the physiological level, which includes special exercises designed mainly to modify the natural faculty of retaining the urethral and anal sphincters.

The spiritual life of the yogi does not at all suppose the total cessation of voluntary sexual activity. There is no opposition between spiritual aspiration and partial abstinence. In fact, rare are the men capable of making the sacrifice involved in total sexual abstinence. Though there are numerous cases of rishis and yogis who are famous for their absolute chastity, many others enter married life generally after practicing chastity during their adolescence.

Aparigraha

Related to *asteya,* this rule aims to regulate the accumulation of riches and possessions of various types in a vain search for happiness. These possessions constitute a source of attachment to the material aspect of our existence, and they are usually not truly indispensable for a healthy life or for a genuine experience of spirituality. Modern people lose a great deal of time seeking riches that are not truly essential. Moreover, safeguarding them often turns into a cause of concern or worry. If we worship what is superfluous, the preservation of what we have acquired results in a loss of precious time and energy, neither of which can be replaced.

The fact of being the privileged owner of material riches is generally associated with attachment, greed, or an insatiable appetite to increase the capital one has amassed. Nevertheless, this rule is not without its exceptions. The possession of riches does not at all exclude the faculty of remaining nonattached and capable of serenely relinquishing them, either on account of circumstances or as a result of a deliberate choice. The momentum of thought can make a prisoner feel more liberated than his jailer, if the latter is the victim of insatiable desires. This sort of nonattachment to earthly goods is found mainly in those who enjoy the rare virtue that is called *vairāgya*. Standing above ordinary states of mind, this yogic nonattachment should not be confused with lack of regard or indifference. It implicitly figures in the famous poem by Rudyard Kipling.

If you can keep your head when all about you
Are losing theirs and blaming it on you;
If you can trust yourself when all men doubt you,
But make allowance for their doubting too;
If you can wait and not be tired by waiting,

Or, being lied about, don't deal in lies,
Or, being hated, don't give way to hating,
And yet don't look too good, nor talk too wise;

If you can dream—and not make dreams your master;
If you can think—and not make thoughts your aim;
If you can meet with triumph and disaster
And treat those two imposters just the same;
If you can bear to hear the truth you've spoken
Twisted by knaves to make a trap for fools,
Or watch the things you gave your life to, broken,
And stoop and build 'em up with worn-out tools;

If you can make one heap of all your winnings
And risk it on one turn of pitch-and-toss,
And lose, and start again at your beginnings
And never breathe a word about your loss;
If you can force your heart and nerve and sinew
To serve your turn long after they are gone,
And so hold on when there is nothing in you
Except the Will which says to them: "Hold on";

If you can talk with crowds and keep your virtue,
Or walk with kings—nor lose the common touch;
If neither foes nor loving friends can hurt you;
If all men count with you, but none too much;
If you can fill the unforgiving minute
With sixty seconds' worth of distance run—
Yours is the Earth and everything that's in it,
*And—which is more—you'll be a Man my son!**

*This version of Kipling's poem reprinted from *A Choice of Kipling's Verse Made by T. S. Eliot* (Scribners, 1943).

5
Niyama—Self-Regulation

The practice of *yama* and *niyama* primarily attracts religious people, regardless of denomination—men and women who have glimpsed, in one way or another, the shadow of their divine nature. But the practice of these ethical rules actually applies to all those who, while aspiring to a healthy, joyful life, realize deep inside that they are already en route, seeking a reality that transcends everyday joys and worries, a timeless reality of truth and love.

While *yama* presents itself as a discipline of behavioral control through its "abstentions," *niyama* concerns the spiritual development of the individual. *Niyama* covers five "observances" directed toward oneself; in other words, they regulate a practitioner's personal conduct.

Śauca

Cleanliness is strongly related to purity, especially in the different disciplines of Yoga. Careful about the elimination of all external and internal body wastes, *śauca* constitutes an important rule in the practice of Haṭha Yoga. External cleanliness of the body is achieved with a hot or cold shower or bath, sweating, exposure to the sun or simply the air, and with massage or friction. Internal cleanliness in Haṭha Yoga is the subject of chapter 9, "*Ṣaṭ Karman*—Purifications."

Santoṣa

Involving a quality of inner equilibrium, *santoṣa* reflects an attitude of contentment that superficially can give the impression of laziness or indeed self-satisfaction, which can be perceived as self-importance, arrogance, or disdain. However, the sought-after state of *santoṣa* is sometimes an extremely positive and dynamic feeling. It is synonymous with inner balance, peace, and imperturbability—not to be confused with passivity. It is an attitude that generates unconditional joy, which is a state of soul that is manifested independently of any external circumstance that the ego views as good news.

Tapas

In Yoga (unlike in the cognitive sciences), especially in the context of Haṭha Yoga, a good understanding of the aims and applications of *tapas* comes from practical experience. The Sanskrit term *tapas* has several meanings and is understood differently according to the practitioner. There being no truly equivalent term, *tapas* is generally translated by "asceticism," a word whose Greek origin denotes exercise. However, the occasionally ambiguous use of the term in yogic doctrine should be noted, as it at times refers to exercise and at other times results. The present exposition does not pretend to go into depth about the origin of yogic asceticism or into its different applications over the centuries. It cannot be exhaustive in the viewpoints and experiences alluded to here.

For the yogi and yogini, *tapas* involves a discipline of austerity as much as purification. In the practice of Haṭha Yoga, this rule aims specifically at mental purification, the development of strength of thought, and endurance. *Tapas* is practiced at three different levels—gentle, medium, and intense. While the first level is relatively accessible to any serious student, the second and third require the guidance of a competent and experienced guru.

The first level may involve different exercises: activating the faculty of empathy, observing strict silence (*mauna*), enduring all kinds of tough weather conditions, experiencing intense heat and cold, and submitting stoically to hunger, thirst, and sleep deprivation. At this level, intense muscular training is proposed, particularly maintaining appropriate postures (*āsanas*) up to the limit of what is tolerable. In the practice of *tapas,* sexual continence can play a significant role, even if at first it is limited to simple control, which consists of abstaining from all sexual thoughts or comments that are out of context. This rule may be accompanied by cutting in half the frequency of sexual activity.*

The path taken (of Yoga *sādhana*) can be favorable for the acquisition of *siddhis,* the superhuman powers to which knowledge and superior states of consciousness are intimately linked. But the *siddhis* a person can acquire on a spiritual journey are still only steps toward the realization of the Self. When the *siddhis* appear, generally at the end of a long quest, the tenacious illusion of the world is set aside, after the practitioner has conscientiously applied the sublime negation of *neti neti* (not this, not that) in each phase of development. Through numerous experiences, the mental world is enriched with new dimensions, notably that of a Reality that eludes the grasp of the mind and the senses. Thenceforth, the perception of the realities of the transitory world only reinforces the practitioners' asceticism and clarifies heightened awareness of the pain and cosmic illusion that surrounds them.

At the end of their spiritual journey, yogis and yoginis are liberated from all the experiences and powers they have acquired during their present lifetime and at the end of numerous past reincarnations. Their liberation, which is for the sole benefit of the Ultimate Reality that is the final objective of all their births, will not exclude the fact of having to immolate what was most sacred to them in the world—the ultimate sacrifice of a spiritual hero—the personal divinity that followed them throughout their quest and to which they were organically attached. Such freedom will be emblematic of the final discharge of all the streams, tributaries, and rivers into the immensity of a vast ocean.

Tapas is emblematic of the spirit of sacrifice, an archetype that is found in many civilizations—a sacrifice that not only allows humans to communicate or commune with the occult forces of nature but also has allowed us to survive during our long evolution on our planet. Dating

*Also see *brahmacarya* in the previous chapter on "*Yama*."

back to ancient times, the term *tapas* figures in hymn X.129 of the *Ṛigveda,* which in its metaphysical description of Creation refers to a heat (*tapas*) emanating from nothing and permitting the appearance of the primordial Being, unmanifested but latent, outside time and space. This term also appears in Patañjali's *Yoga Sūtras* (IV.1), in which he describes one of the paths leading to the acquisition of extraordinary powers (*siddhis*), along with four other considerations (birth, certain herbal beverages, *mantras,* and *samādhi*). The text lists about thirty such powers.

These superhuman powers are acquired by beings who live for the most part in great destitution and near absolute anonymity. In India they are considered as enduring heroes and, for a long time, have constituted the spiritual leaders of an elite asceticism. Their mental universe is located beyond the noisy world, the newsworthy events in society, far from the gaze of the ephemeral protagonists in political or social power, in sport or show business. Extreme practices rest on an unshakeable faith, anchored in a cultural environment that seems to defy the laws of time. Anonymous champions of determination and psychic force, this spiritual elite demonstrates an exceptional will and stamina. Their powers are often accompanied by universal compassion and immeasurable patience, which are the conditions for grace to descend and crown these unconditional lovers of God.

The most visible superhuman exploits are seen among the *sādhus* and the *naga nagas* or *naga babas,* whose principal feature is total nudity; they pour regularly out of the four corners of India, principally the Himalayas where they live as hermits or anchorites. They come down from their hermitages or lonely huts to the banks of the Ganges to participate in great traditional gatherings (*melas*), which in India take place every four years in rotation in four different towns: Nasik, Ujjain, Allahabad, and Hardwar. Received everywhere with reverence and devotion, those who possess *siddhi* powers enjoy great respect from their peers, from Indian civil and military dignitaries, as well as from the mass of pilgrims who sometimes number in the millions. This highly colorful crowd is united in contemplation and meditation and also in what it considers to be the privilege of *darśana,* the vision of these exemplary beings who bear a universal blessing. For this multitude, composed of ethnic groups with very different languages and coming from diverse social milieus and castes, the *naga nagas* become a living source of emulation, a model of the faith that moves mountains and orients the hearts of the believers toward Heaven.

Coming from a very ancient spiritual school, reputedly atypical because of its adepts' heterodox behavior, these extreme ascetics have renounced all worldly goods. In the vast Indian continent, one is used to hearing: "If it doesn't exist in India, it doesn't exist anywhere." It is therefore not a paradox to see men, for the most part entirely nude, move around freely, without risk of opprobrium for indecency, while Bharata (India), "the largest democracy in the world," typically displays, even today, a Victorian sense of modesty and fear of promiscuity. Still, with the exception of a minority of Hindu purists who are strictly faithful to the precept according to which the yogi must never make a display of his spirituality, and who thus scarcely appreciate these public events, the *naga naga* elicit amazement and admiration. They are exceptional beings who are treated with respect mixed with fear because, according to popular legend, those who possess *siddhis* can be dangerous when angered.

It is equally possible to witness the demonstration of certain forms of *siddhis* in public places in India. These are "fallen" yogis who have decided deliberately to ignore the fact that it is attachment to extraordinary powers that precipitates their fall and that only the condition of nonattachment will allow them to attain the ultimate Reality. These Yoga renegades are victims in the grip of an extraordinary power, who have renounced the path of a challenging spiritual quest, preferring instead to attract crowds by virtue of their "magical" powers. From the strict point of view of the *sādhana,* the status of yogi is then replaced by that of *fakir,* an Arabic word meaning "poor person" (beggar).

Svādhyāya

Quite as important at the level of knowledge is the rule designated by the term *svādhyāya,* which recommends the study of sacred texts. If it is indispensable to acquire basic training in the practical study of any science, it is all the more desirable for every believer to study the foundations of his or her own religion. In the same way, the atheist, who does not deny the necessity of rules to manage life in society and who thus adheres to its values, will have everything to gain by knowing the rules that this same society imposes while granting freedom of thought.

Without study of sacred writings and, of course, putting them into practice, religion risks becoming the source of intolerance and, alas, bloody conflicts. Dogmatic practices can also result in the cult of superstition, robotic orthodoxy, and isolation of the individual in a cultural and social no-man's-land. In the spirit of Haṭha Yoga, recommended study includes the sacred texts belonging to each person's confession, whether it is the Gospels, the Qur'an, or the Torah, or Indian sacred scriptures. More than a source of strictly theological or philosophical knowledge, the study aimed at in the practice of *svādhyāya* is, for the Haṭha yogi, a source of emotional inspiration and meditation.

Nevertheless, in a universal context of a spirituality excluding prejudice and narrow-mindedness, the yogi can just as easily find refuge and emulation at the heart of other sources of spiritual inspiration. Thus it is that the famous nineteenth-century Indian yogi Sri Ramakrishna experienced repeated unions with the Divine triggered by sublime inspirations found as much in the reading of the Qur'an or the Bible as in the writings of his own tradition. The study required by *svādhyāya* also includes *japa,* repetition of the *mantra* that usually completes the traditional initiation of the *cela* (student) by his or her guru.

Īśvarapraṇidhāna

The last of the ten fundamental rules of Haṭha Yoga, the highly religious *īśvarapraṇidhāna* is not the least important. In fact, it presupposes a sincere and intense devotion, a reorientation of thought and feeling toward the Absolute, the goal of all spirituality. From the technical point of view, it consists of a state of divinely inspired mental concentration directed exclusively toward the Divine, Īśvara, the Lord who is none other than the supreme awareness of the Self. Īśvara is different from the Creator God of the Judeo-Christian tradition insofar as Īśvara is the transcendent awareness of the Self, free from ontological illusion and, consequently, of all spatiotemporal or cognitive dependency.

The yogi's progress on the long spiritual journey that leads to a determined return to the source involves deliberately abandoning the self to the Beloved, to the Divine, and to the unknown designs of immanent Will, with the hope of one day becoming its very humble instrument. This done, the yogi places himself or herself at the heart of Bhakti Yoga (the Yoga of devotion), at the heart of Divine love.

6
Āsanas—Postures

Āsanas, the third part of Haṭha Yoga, are today a victim, either from ignorance or a concern for simplification, of an unfortunate conflation that tarnishes the whole teaching of Yoga by reducing it to yogic postures. Under cover of educational or therapeutic intentions, this reductionist notion, always arbitrary and often opportunistic, and with a mercenary aim, explains to a great degree the abundance of methods offered to the general public.

It is, above all, in the Western world that we find the misappropriation of the empirical tradition of these intangible resources, whose ancient origins and sacred character welcome everyone, and yet at times become the prey of ignorant or time-serving, dishonest individuals. These people do not hesitate a single moment to formally establish an exclusive right to market their services via millennium-old words such as *mantra,* often with unaware public institutions, thereby preventing a continued good faith use by others. There are also cases of patent rights' claims for traditional *āsanas,* or particular series of *āsanas,* where smart business-minded applicants invoke a personal style to justify their senseless claims.

Other than certain methods and techniques transmitted orally by highly responsible yogis, a number of discoveries of the yogic heritage are available to whoever wishes to appropriate, transform, and exploit them. The goal of the monopolization of the yogic patrimony, often under the label "amateur/imitator," is for the most part lucrative, when it does not serve the vain self-glorification of an "illumined" initiator or founder of a self-proclaimed sect. While such appropriations are doubtless legal, they remain nevertheless ethically debatable. Unaware, or feigning unawareness, of the yogic origin of the new product they are commercializing, the appropriators refrain from mentioning the original source of the service they are marketing to the general public. Only respect and a deep study of the sacred nature of the origins of Yoga will lead to a decent restraint in its dissemination.

In a world that favors miracle cures and fast money to the detriment of serious study and the search for durable ethical values, Yoga is presented in a superficial way. Among the many derivatives of Yoga, we should note the artistic sport of "calisthenics," the self-control method of Coué, Pilates, energy manipulation in Japanese Reiki, and sophrology, without forgetting an impressive range of exercises for relaxation and "meditation" offered by many medical or educational institutions, or even spas as a common service along with other beauty treatments. On a strictly physical level, we should mention stretching techniques, "aerobics," and other fitness fads of the day. It is also in the vast repertoire of Yoga that visualization and mental exercises are found, the ones so esteemed by coaches of high-level sportsmen, business leaders, and other persons in charge of the industrial and commercial world.

As a result of its unlimited availability in a world that is hardly eager to respect what seems to it to be an unhoped-for windfall for enriching itself, the doctrine of Yoga also feeds the imaginary world inhabited by the promoters of new sectarian ideologies. These are generally based on arbitrary and ignorant interpretations of its sacred nature. Their objectives are sometimes doubtful, and even abusive. They are directed at a category of people who are easily duped by these unscrupulous predators, often with harmful social consequences.

The production of both physical and mental effort allows a person to extract from Yoga the energy that will bring a beneficial feeling of self-control, well-being, virtue (from the Latin *virtus,* "a valorous man, aware of his force"), and the enjoyable pleasure that is obtained when the will is exercised. In the spirit of traditional Haṭha Yoga, which rests on the ten ethical rules of *yama* and *niyama,* such self-assertion or efficiency in action—something that in principle could help criminal persons in being more "efficient" in their wrongdoings—has no relationship with self-assertiveness or Nietzsche's ideal of the superman. This is because, even though the yogi is fully invested in a supreme effort to achieve physical perfection, such a person's gaze is not lowered, like that of a predator; it is raised, on the contrary, toward an elevated ideal, yet without ignoring the surrounding world or its distress.

Rather than acting directly on the mind, as does Raja Yoga, Haṭ ha Yoga presents the idea that the mind can be reached and influenced through physical exercise, and more particularly through the exercise of voluntary muscles. Motions are achieved at the gross muscular level after their natural beginning as fine, downward oscillations of the mind.

At different levels of its practice, such as in Jala Vasti or Vajrolī, Haṭha Yoga teaches methods that aim at reversing the body's constant tendency to downward motion. To achieve such reverse motions supposes, however, a perfect technique, much practice, determination, and perseverance. In harnessing these motions along with the mental oscillations, *āsanas* are the first step toward preliminary mind control while providing *sukha* (ease) and *sthira* (calmness).

There is no clear and definite information on the number of existing *āsanas*. Hindu tradition claims eighty-four thousand, while the *Haṭha Yoga Pradīpikā,* an old basic text on Haṭha Yoga, refers to eighty-four *āsanas,* mentioning only a few by name. Sri S. S. Goswami illustrates his classic manual *Advanced Haṭha Yoga* with 108 *āsanas,* and is thus at variance with other contemporary authors who include many *āsana* variants in their counting. Innumerable as they are, the *āsanas* are intended to influence the innumerable thought-patterns.

The arbitrarily selected sample of *āsanas* displayed in the color plates, which are performed in the Goswami Yoga style, demonstrate how Haṭha Yoga can aid the development of a symmetrical and well-controlled body. Besides some speculative interpretations of the aesthetics and ethics of *āsanas,* it remains a fact that in yogic tradition these psychophysical performances carry the dedicated efforts of would-be yogis toward a higher spiritual ideal. *Āsanas* may also be regarded as willful acts intended to bring forth control and harmony and elevate consciousness above the sensorial. They are the tangible cornerstone of a spiritual culture that aims at developing a well-controlled body, vitalized and purified by various cleaning methods, yogic asceticism (*tapas*), and the application of ethical rules, *yama* and *niyama*. Spiritually empowered and equipped with a flexible and strong body, the adept is then able to endure life's inescapable crises and the challenges of *sādhana*.

Too often, today's practice and obtuse interpretations of Haṭha Yoga *āsanas* are the repository of deep misunderstandings about the role and aims of the third limb of Aṣṭānga Yoga. Analytical points of view emphasizing the alleged benefits of specific postures—often in comparison to other physical exercises, gymnastics, fitness, and aerobics—are not relevant for a yogic discipline with a vocation that is fundamentally holistic.

It is, of course, indisputable that a regular practice of certain *āsanas* may strengthen the body, make it more supple, enduring, and often even release a temporary sense of well-being. But the so-often-sought feel-good effects or excitement resulting from Haṭha Yoga workouts do not really go beyond the realm of the individual, with highly subjective, temporary sensations, added to which wishful thinking as placebo often plays an important role. To be wise and hopefully find a way to achieve durable results, it is far better to place oneself and one's efforts in the right context from the outset, remembering that *āsanas* are no panacea per se. What is good for one person may turn out to be risky or quite inappropriate for another.

To objectively assess the merits and value of *āsana* training, it is therefore important to refrain from speculating too much, dissecting or generalizing on the basis of the benefits of one or two specific *āsanas*. In the Haṭha Yoga practice, as elsewhere, certain prerequisites are to be taken into account. After all, training conditions vary according to the individual's age, personal ambitions, motivation depth, health condition, and, last but not least, the time available for training, which is crucial, given that success is intimately bound to regularity in exercise.

As regards the other party of the "partnership," the teaching proper, it is important to remember that genuine, traditional Yoga teaching supposes high credentials, something that is often ignored in the West. I still remember Ma Santi Devi saying: "Nowadays, there are more gurus than genuine *celas*!"

As with school education, and perhaps still more when it comes to the practice of Yoga, the presence of a teacher who is unselfish, knowledgeable, and experienced is really a must. As with Aristotle's formula "*logos, pathos, ethos,*" given when he was advising would-be experts in the art of politics, to properly conduct an *āsana* class, it is not sufficient to just enumerate the *āsanas* to be executed one after another. This is no more than the first step of an enriching lesson.

More complete than any other athletic discipline, the *āsanas* simultaneously include force, flexibility, speed, and endurance. A regular practice of Haṭha Yoga makes it possible to model one's body upon a harmonious symmetry of proportions, to increase energy, to balance it, and to make it capable of effort. To do this, it is essential to methodically practice various exercises of relaxation and mental concentration. Over time, the practice of *āsanas* has evolved considerably. It has become a method that is perfectly adapted to the needs of modern people. It includes dynamic and static exercises as well as a complementary method of muscular contractions (detailed in the next chapter, "*Cāraṇā*—Yogic Bodybuilding").

Though it is true that *āsanas* are very important in the practice of Haṭha Yoga, it is also the case that their effectiveness is apparent only when they are practiced intelligently, preferably regularly with other complementary disciplines, particularly purifying acts (*ṣaṭ karman*), control of the life force (*prāṇāyāma*), and mental concentration.

The importance of these notably psychophysical exercises has not escaped the notice of Indian sages, which is why most ancient writings repeatedly recommend mastery of the body. In fact, all Yoga schools, whether Mantra Yoga, Laya Yoga, or Raja Yoga, suppose that the meditator has gained control of the seated posture, generally with legs crossed and the spine kept perfectly straight. Thus the text *Vedāntadarśana* (4.1.9) states: "Mental concentration depends on an unmoving (straight) body posture."

The term *āsana* is very ancient. It is found in the Veda Samhītās and also the Brāhmaṇas. It was the god Śiva who revealed the processes of the manifold types of *āsanas,* thus demonstrating their pre-Upaniṣad origins. However, the sage Patañjali was the first to describe their technical value by introducing them in the eightfold path of Yoga (Aṣṭānga Yoga).

The root of the word, *āsa* or *as,* indicates a motionless physical state. *Āsanas* are thus traditionally static postures. Their application involves two distinct methods: a static phase facilitating the practice of mental concentration and a dynamic phase that serves as preparation for the static phase. The static phase of an *āsana,* that is to say, the maintenance of a suitable unmoving posture, requires a certain preparation, in particular the practice of synchronized movements in a starting posture, "A," which evolves into another posture, "B." In the execution of these movements, breathing is rhythmic, the body relaxed, and attention fully mobilized. The dynamic application of *āsanas* is always preliminary to that of a static *āsana*. The former has in particular the effect of countering the prolonged muscular inactivity of the latter.

Static Exercises

In Haṭha Yoga, methods have been conceived to create concentration postures that provide a good base for the student, while procuring a feeling of ease. These methods are termed static or isometric exercises, and they require maintaining certain special positions for a particular period of time. Three phases are distinguished during the training: easy, painful, and a phase of willpower.

The easy phase has the feature of being free of any discomfort. A degree of training in this phase supports serenity and powers of concentration. Physically, this implies that the body can function without impediment. The vital functions become stronger, which leads to better health. The goal of Haṭha Yoga is, as a result of the static exercises, to combine the best physical and mental conditions in order to reach an optimal state of concentration, as well as better health.

The easy phase is followed by a painful phase, which follows a preliminary phase of discomfort. Training makes it possible to acquire the capacity to endure the pain. In this way endurance increases and the immune system is boosted.

The third phase starts when the pain becomes almost unbearable. The capacity to endure the pain, developed by a special method of concentration, greatly contributes to the reinforcement of the will. When this method is practiced in a state of breath suspension, the effect is further amplified. The phase of willpower is then reached. Finally, the moment arrives when the pain becomes absolutely unbearable, and the maintenance of the posture must be stopped. In regular training, it is not advisable to continue beyond the first feeling of discomfort. The transition to the phases of pain and willpower must be accomplished gradually and under the supervision of a qualified teacher.

Every part of the body is reinforced by static exercises. The back, the abdomen, and the pelvis are trained to remain absolutely unmoving. Included in these exercises are the reversed postures, standing on the head or the shoulders. In addition to their contribution to mental concentration, static exercises have no equal for developing endurance, invigorating the nervous system, and contributing to optimal health.

Dynamic Exercises

In order to carry out the static exercises in the most effective and beneficial way possible, dynamic exercises are an essential preliminary preparation; they facilitate control of the muscles, making them flexible, strong, and able to tolerate strain. The dynamic exercises are postural movements that, practiced methodically, promote good muscular development. The mental concentration exerted on the muscles and with the movements plays a very important part. A static posture can be successful only if it is supported by its dynamic version.

The dynamic exercises are grouped into six categories—dorsal, abdominal, pelvic, neck, arms, legs—with the aim of developing the principal groups of muscles, that is, the dorsal, abdominal, and respiratory (thoracic and diaphragm). The training of the leg muscles aims at optimizing the activity of the dorsal and abdominal muscles. Complementary exercises have been created for that purpose.

Āsanas (postures) and *cāraṇā* (exercises of contraction and muscular control) introduce the first stage of exercises combined with concentration. They consist of front, back, and side flexions, torsions, extensions of the limbs outward and backward, pendulum and rotational movements. The ancient system of gymnastics for girls, known as "calisthenics" (general balance movements on the head or shoulders), as well as the modern exercises of muscular control, all have their origin in *āsanas* and *cāraṇā*.

The movements are based on two fundamental principles: the choice of a posture appropriate to the desired effect and the progressive adaptation to the movements. In the discipline of Haṭha Yoga, a given posture allows the contraction and the extension of the muscles to be light, medium, or strong. Thus the postures are classified into light, medium, or strong contractions. According to the muscular development of the pupil, a posture is selected from one of these alternatives.

7

Cāraṇā–Yogic Bodybuilding

Advanced muscular control has been known in India for millennia. Among Haṭha Yoga's training methods, there is one form of muscular control, *cāraṇā,* which consists of a threefold training process. In targeting specific muscles, this particular training requires elementary body awareness, as it targets specific muscles or groups of muscles, while other "antagonistic" muscles are to be kept quite relaxed; it also requires maximum willpower in the muscle contraction and a breathing rhythm that is designed according to the exercises. It additionally supposes the faculty to quickly and fully relax the muscles during the short intervals between two consecutive muscle contractions.

Cāraṇā comprises both dynamic and static exercises, and the goal is to produce a certain type of movement where voluntary contraction is as predominant as muscular control. This control is exerted equally on the principal and secondary muscles. *Cāraṇā* complements the practice of the *āsanas* by hardening the musculature and by developing mental concentration.

At an advanced stage, the main goal of this type of exercise is to develop mental concentration on striated muscles until one can control the smooth muscles. When the muscles are thus perfectly controlled, it becomes possible to influence the activity of the internal organs in order to achieve particular aims. This yogic method fully develops the capacity of the abdominal muscles and the pelvis to influence the work of the digestive and genital systems. The system of contraction and muscular control includes contraction and control exercises, abdominal control, and pelvic control.

Contraction and Control Exercises

In Haṭha Yoga, *cāraṇā* consists mainly of natural movements carried out by a voluntary contraction that is always controlled. When a person is mentally assured of muscular control, it becomes possible to control one or more groups of muscles at the same time, to contract all the muscles of the body, or to slacken the whole body or only certain parts of it. *Cāraṇā* consists primarily of the following exercises:

1. Griva Cāraṇā (Movements of the Neck), which include:
   a. Forward flexion, extension, lateral flexion, and rotation of the head with voluntary contraction
   b. Voluntary control of the orofacial muscle (subcutaneous muscle) and of the sternocleidomastoid muscle (nodding movement)
2. Udara Cāraṇā (Movements of the Abdominal Muscles) including:
   a. Flexion, extension, and lateral flexion of the trunk, and rotational movements, all carried out with voluntary contractions
   b. Flexion of the hips
   c. Voluntary movements of the abdominal muscles, which involve the practice of an important exercise of control, Tounda Cālaṇā, which is divided into three parts:
      - Voluntary distension of only the higher part of the abdomen
      - Voluntary distension of only the lower part
      - Wave movement from top to bottom of the abdominal wall while it is retracted
3. Bahu Cāraṇā (Movements of the Arms) including:
   a. Adductor movements of the shoulders upward, downward, forward, and backward

b. Flexion and extension of the arms, adductor movements of the arms outward and back, rocking movements, and rotation of the arms
c. Flexion, extension, and posterior-anterior rotation backward and forward toward the front of the forearms
d. Flexion and extension of the hands, rotation with the palms forward and backward, circular motions
e. Flexion and extension of the fingers with voluntary contractions
f. Movements controlled by the pectorals, serratus major, dorsal, scapulas, trapezoids, deltoids, biceps, triceps, and muscles of contraction and extension of the forearm

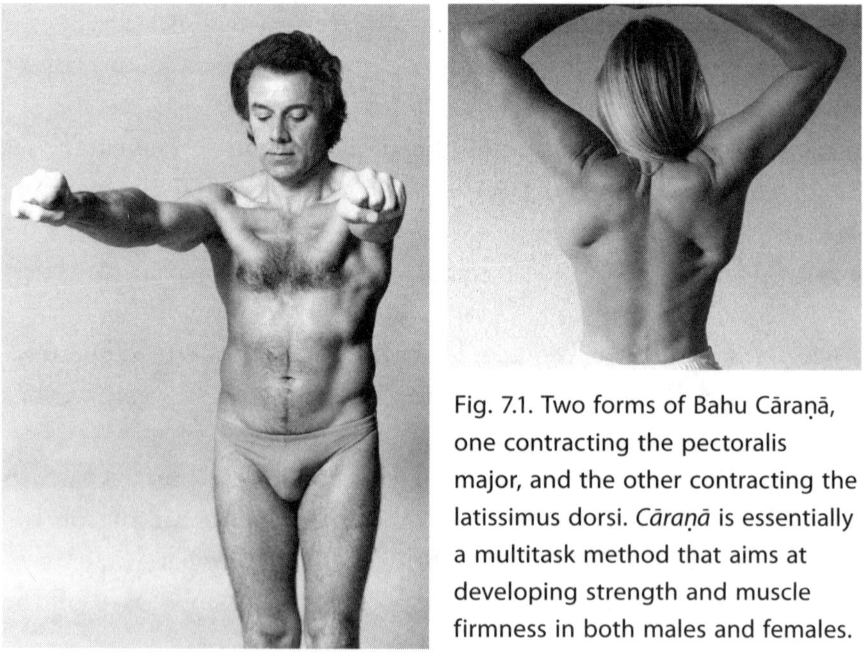

Fig. 7.1. Two forms of Bahu Cāraṇā, one contracting the pectoralis major, and the other contracting the latissimus dorsi. *Cāraṇā* is essentially a multitask method that aims at developing strength and muscle firmness in both males and females.

4. Śakti Cāraṇā (Movements of the Legs), including:
   a. On the level of the hip, flexion, extension, balance, and rotational movements
   b. Flexion and extension of the leg
   c. Flexion and extension of the foot

d. Flexion and extension of the toes, rotation in both directions, all movements being carried out with voluntary contractions
e. Controlled movements of the thigh and the calf muscles

Abdominal Control

This includes three principal exercises: Agnisāra (Abdominal Retraction and Release), Uḍḍīyāna (Abdominal Retraction), and Naulī (Straight Muscle Exercise).

Agnisāra consists of a fast succession of alternating retractions and relaxations of the abdominal wall, carried out in a state of apnea (suspended breath) following expiration.

Uḍḍīyāna consists of maximally retracting the abdominal wall inward and upward for a given amount of time, in a state of apnea (suspended breath) following expiration.

Naulī constitutes the highest degree of abdominal control. The principal phases of this exercise consist of the central isolation of the rectus abdominis, lateral isolation, right and left, the isolation on the right-hand side of both recti and the same on the left side, while passing alternately from the right contraction to the left contraction of the rectus abdominis and, finally, a side movement with the help of this muscle (see fig. 9.2).

At an advanced stage of control of the abdomen, it is also possible to isolate the two semilunaris (sinews) separately, together, and even simultaneously to join them together with the rectus abdominis (see fig. 9.4).

Pelvic Control

These movements aim to reinforce and control the muscles and organs of the pelvis. Two important exercises are involved. The first, Aśvinī Mudrā (Dynamic Anal Control), consists of a contraction alternating with the relaxation of the anal sphincters, whereas the second, Mūla Bandha (Static Anal Control), is a contraction maintained for a given time. At a more advanced stage, these exercises are practiced with abdominal control and *prāṇāyāma*. These exercises reinforce sexual power and the control of impulses.

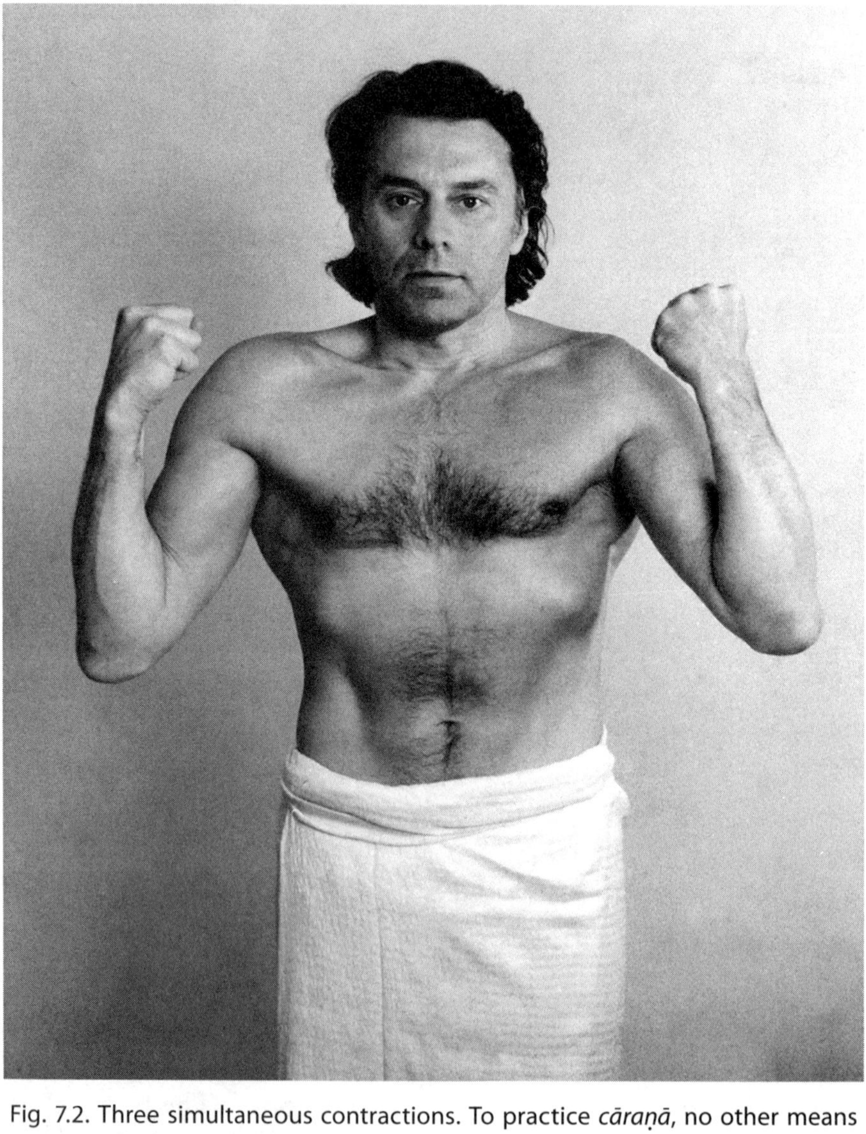

Fig. 7.2. Three simultaneous contractions. To practice *cāraṇā*, no other means are required than well-developed body awareness and the power to fully concentrate the will to achieve maximum contraction and then relaxation of specific muscles or groups of muscles.

Mudrās, Exercises of Control

The very ancient term *mudrā*, mentioned in the Brāhmaṇas, Upaniṣ. ads, and Tantras, is subject to two technical interpretations: it indicates either the gestural postures of the fingers or hand, or the exercises of specific muscular contractions. The first category of *mudrās* is most often used in the practice of Mantra Yoga. The second is in fact a constituent part of Haṭha Yoga, and the *mudrās* overlap with *cāraṇā*.

Similar but distinct from the *āsanas* that they complement, the *mudrās* are postural, exercises that are integrated into the rewarding path of Haṭha Yoga. A *mudrā* is practiced during an *āsana* or independently, in the form of static postures or movements. It consists mainly of the control of the contraction of certain muscles, which can be accompanied by specific respiratory methods.

Frequently quoted in the literature on the Upaniṣads, *mudrās* are recommended to the Yoga practitioner on account of their purifying effects. For example, the Mahā Mudrā is well known for its beneficial influence on the two phases of metabolism. Of about a hundred *mudrās* that are actually mentioned in the literature, only a few are taught. Among the most frequent coming from the teaching of contemporary Haṭha Yoga, the following deserve mention:

- Jālandhara Bandha, Chin Lock (muscular contraction of the nape of the neck)
- Uḍḍīyāna Bandha, Abdominal Retraction (during breath suspension)
- Mahā Bandha or Mahā Mudrā, Great Lock (anaerobic posture)
- Viparītakaraṇī, Modified Shoulder Stand (posture on the shoulders)
- Khecarī Mudrā, Advanced Breath Suspension (closure of the glottis by lingual introversion)

There are other *mudrās* used in advanced exercises, like Sahajolī, Amarolī, and Vajrolī. At various levels they play a paramount part in the control of the body and mind, as well as in their protection. Here control or mastery means the conscious application of the will in order to modify—in the form of hyperactivity, hypoactivity, inversion, or cessation—the normal function of an organ or of the skeletal muscles. Sahajolī and Amarolī are used more commonly, as Vajrolī in most cases presents serious difficulties for the practitioner.

Sahajolī is an exercise that primarily consists in practicing Yoni Mudrā in association with pelvic exercises. Amarolī is a specific method of various applications of one's own urine. Within the framework of Yoga, this method is closely related to the pelvic exercises mentioned above, which are complementary to it. Amarolī is in fact an ancient organ therapy mentioned in Ayurvedic literature and also explained in the Bible. Esteemed by the *naga sāddhus* and Tibetan monks, the technique is practiced with one's own urine, which can be ingested, used for massage, or drawn in through the nasal passages. This natural "organotherapy" drew international attention when one of its famous followers, Sri Morarji Desai, former Prime Minister of India, wrote a book on its benefits. It is also relevant here to mention Sarasvatī Cālana, an important *mudrā* on the path of awakening and the progression of the Kuṇḍalinī energy.

In Haṭha Yoga the natural downward peristalsis movements resulting from sexual thought and emotion can be neutralized by the methodically applied technique of Vajrolī, in which self-control goes to a higher level. The exercise aims at the maximum effectiveness of the sexual organs, together with total mastery of them. Practiced in successive stages, it is the prerogative of advanced followers of Yoga. For the yogi, it is in particular a question of learning the difficult art of absorbing atmospheric air and liquids into his bladder, by way of the urethra, and then expelling them by the same way. This rare yogic control of the urethra was presented to the medical profession at the time of Sri S. S. Goswami's world tour of New York, Tokyo, Paris, and Stockholm by his close disciple, the Haṭha yogi Dr. Dinabandhu Pramanick.

8
Yogic Sexual Mastery

Sexual energy, which is an immanent natural power and essential for the reproduction of the species, plays a paramount part in the maintenance of all organic life on our planet. It is, according to the doctrines of Yoga, a specific effect of the vital force (*prāṇa*). This sexual energy and its interaction with health and longevity did not escape the lucid observations and daring experiments of Indian sages. Their thorough study of the subject, corroborated by empirical knowledge, gave a new dimension to this incontrovertible phenomenon of human life.

Particularly for men, the sexual instinct is probably the most difficult force to dominate. Wise Hindus have long noted that beliefs, reprimands, or even spontaneous mortifications do not have any lasting effect, that they constitute at best a momentary diversion of generally irrepressible impulses. Just as rishis and yogis of old could reveal to *Homo sapiens* a new mental dimension (*turīya*) in addition to our three current states of consciousness—waking, sleeping, dreaming—the daring pioneers of mental introspection revealed to the world the fourth dimension of sexuality, which goes beyond the stages of growth, procreation, and pleasure.

The description of this dimension often refers to a metaphysical causality, such as the subtle world of the vital force (*prāṇa vāyu*), which forms a bridge between the body and the mind. Once mastered, this force allows a couple, in a free and harmonious union, to go beyond the limits of sensual pleasure (*bhoga*), specific abstinence (*brahmacharya*), or *coitus reservatus* or *interruptus,* if desired. In the Tantric tradition, sexual energy is not used to reach the height of pleasure in a vain explosion of ecstasy. It is used with the sacred vision of an effective transmutation of the ego into a reality that transcends it.

Paradoxically, although there have been many incursions into and borrowings from the Tantric literature, this fourth dimension of sexuality seems to have escaped the attention of modern humanity, despite the greed for knowledge. The reason is undoubtedly the new paradigm that it introduces, as well as the subtle technique of this universal force, most often transmitted orally or in the form of rare writings. Its highly technical nature makes it impenetrable to the modern world on account of a lack of cultural correspondences.

The control of sexual energy is mentioned in the *Ṛigveda*. According to the *Yogatattvopaniṣad,* the adamantine method of Vajrolī Mudrā, derived from *brahmacarya,* plays a paramount role in the control of sexuality. It has the effect of turning a practitioner into an accomplished yogi. Its specific goal is nothing less than to overcome sexual energy through various processes in which the yogi passes through the whole phenomenon of sexuality in its psychological, emotional, organic, glandular, and muscular phases. When the yogi faithfully carries out this ancient method, which is generally reserved for exceptional practitioners, he crosses the virtual barrier that leads him from Haṭha Yoga into the realm of higher-level mastery—Raja Yoga.

Before attaining the control that allows the suction of air or liquids through the urethra, the yogi will most certainly have already practiced Aśvinī Mudrā regularly, alternating contractions with relaxation of the anus to culminate in Mūla Bandha, which consists of a firmly maintained maximal contraction. He will then have recourse to the method of Linga Śankocana, which *Dhyānabindopaniṣad* explicitly envisages as an alternating movement of the penis in the form of a retraction inside the body followed by an extension toward the outside. These acts of preliminary control will then allow him, using Yoni Mudrā, to use *prāṇāyāmic* force to bring back into his own body, via urethral suction, the sperm previously deposited into the vagina of the yogini.

Sexual Fusion

The advanced exercises of sexual control are explicitly described in the Upaniṣads. In this context seminal energy is indicated by the term *ojas,* and its function consists in invigorating the whole body and prolonging human life. With the assistance of Yoni Mudrā, a yogi and yogini can control their sexuality, initially individually and later together, while accurately following the instructions of a guru who is an expert in the field.

Followers of this spiritual practice of sexual fusion are young people, generally under thirty years of age. They have a spiritual dimension that is often accompanied by a well-developed sexuality. Endowed with exceptional strength, these followers of the purest Tantric art do not use aphrodisiacs, which are products designed to stimulate the libido and achieve desire. Stimulation for these lovers of the spiritual life depends mostly on the strong attraction that they experience for each other.

Thus a man can maintain coitus without interruption for five hours with a maximum of two ejaculations, at the beginning and the end. He can also have three to five consecutive ejaculations, with a brief interval of one to two minutes, without ever separating from his partner, or he can make the coupling last for a period of one and a half to two hours, with only one ejaculation at the end of the session.

His partner, who is qualified and specially chosen for this very unusual union, will be able to maintain sexual union for up to five hours at a stretch, delay for a long time the release of her orgasm during the course of a very extended coupling, or enjoy ten consecutive orgasms or more, in one single prolonged union. These Tantric practices, characterized by a remarkable control and a superior harmony, have no reported side effects to my knowledge.

Although these acts of control of sexual energy can today appear very difficult, if not impossible, for modern people to accomplish, nevertheless they unquestionably open extremely interesting perspectives, *mutatis mutandis,* on human potential in general and on the question of contraception (a natural aspect of these techniques) in particular, for a planet undergoing a population explosion.

The Five "M"s

It goes without saying that the Vajrolī method is particularly difficult to master. A Tantric method exists, however, which can be substituted and is relatively more accessible. This is *pañca makāra,* the process of the five "M"s. Although it is not inherent in traditional Haṭha Yoga (see however the rule of *brahmacarya*), the secret Tantric rite of the five "M"s (in Hinduism and later in Tibetan Buddhism) illustrates the awakening of the dependence of the senses on their object, in particular the hold exerted by sexuality, while realizing the possibility of its control in a spiritual context.

Applying to both men and women, sexual control means here the control of thought, emotion, and action. It is extremely difficult to control the thinking and emotional processes by merely applying determination and will, but yogic experiences clearly indicate that thought and emotional control is comparatively easier through first learning control in regards to the physical object of desire. The five "M"s (*pañca makāra*) are the initials of the Sanskrit words *madhya* (wines and spirits), *matsya* (fish), *māmasa* (meat), *mudrā* (dried pulses), *maithuna* (sexual union). Supposed aphrodisiacs, these foodstuffs and the act that accompanies them are generally not recommended for the Hindu faithful.

Certain Tantric schools give a purely symbolic interpretation of this rite by substituting other terms for those enumerated above. Sexual union is replaced by a floral offering, received by hands forming the tortoise *mudrā*. In both cases, however, it relates to a spiritual discipline that aims at transcending the play of polarities of the mind (*rāga-dveṣa*).

Whether they are of Hindu or Tibetan origin, the writings devoted to the rite of the five "M"s suppose adequate skill (*adhikāra*) on the part of the reader. Candidates for this Tantric process must be suitable on the physical, social, mental, and moral planes. As a result, the *Kularnava Tantra* excludes the glutton, libertine, cynic, miser, ignoramus, hypocrite, and drunkard, whereas the *Gautamiya Tantra* admits those who have conquered passion, indolence, illusory knowledge, and anger. In the same spirit, the *Gandharva Tantra* requires the applicant to be pure and believing, intelligent, master of the senses, abstain from any violence toward any creature, and a performer of good actions toward others. The various Tantric schools generally make faith in God a condition sine qua non for the practice of the five "M"s.

The necessary purity is described by the key term *śukra,* appearing in Āyurveda, the Brāhmaṇas, and in particular three Upaniṣads, in which we can read: "Just as the Supreme Being is pure, *śukra* is pure." There is no equivalent in the West, but the conception and perception of this purity are the support of all sexuality, the source of every sexual characteristic, the physiology of male and female genitals.

Śukra, the principle of sexuality, originates in the primordial Śakti, which supports Brahman (Supreme Consciousness) and is the one reality within a formless infinity. This Śakti is also a superpower (*vibhūti*) that is latent on the level of the Infinite and is activated when the Infinite is veiled. And yet, it is precisely this veil that constitutes the universe and its forms, a universe that is really not deprived of sense, real as it is in its pragmatism, even if it rests on a transcendent reality.

When the *vibhūti* of Śakti manifests its very first form, it is in fact the manifestation of *śukra* (*Guhya-Kālyopaniṣad*, 52), although any sexual desire is absent at this stage. This first manifestation is *śukra* personified—the Divine Mother. Whoever is aware of it will be beyond the sexual influence of *śukra* (*Muṇḍakopaniṣad*, 3.2.1) and will then be able to sing the *mantra*: *"Om śukrāya svaha"* (*Vanadurgopaniṣad*).

The pleasure of two lovers whose passion bursts into a harmonious union can surely be regarded as a beautiful pagan sacrament, a blind call toward the Absolute. But in the Tantric space, the seemingly similar body-and-soul union of a spiritually attuned couple escapes both morality, as commonly perceived, and rational judgment. It exhibits, though, the less known fourth dimension of sexual power—a contribution to humankind almost as valuable as the yogic discovery of mind's fourth dimension of *turīya,* which illustrates spiritual awakening.

The rules of admission are strict for candidates wishing to practice the five "M"s. They apply only to those who are ready to follow a path that from time immemorial has been regarded as dangerous and difficult, and demanding in terms of personal sacrifices. The practitioner who has succeeded in qualifying is described as a *vīra* (hero). He will obey flawlessly (tradition obliges him) every instruction of his guru.

The basis for the practice of *maithuna* (sexual intercourse) consists of a couple composed of two disciples (*śiṣya*) of opposite sex, who are prepared beforehand by their spiritual master. The couple then penetrates into a world of realities sometimes considered very unorthodox by society. Seen from the outside, they will probably be regarded as a couple of hedonists who dare to disregard morality and disdain traditional taboos. In fact, this atypical couple will endeavor to transcend the dualistic energy of desire, *rāga,* which is the source of sensual pleasure, and its opposite, *dveṣa*. These special lovers of spirituality will then have to rise up, sublimate their feelings, and transform the profane into the sacred. The inspirational grandeur and beauty of those special athletes of Eros struggling on a two-edged path is really in line with the yogic *deva deha* ideal of excellence. Such a unique metamorphosis needs its poet or a master in lyrics to be described adequately.

The yogini in such a couple conforms to certain specific selection criteria; she has been individually trained, and in every way has the same status as her partner as she completely shares his spiritual aspirations. It should be noted that women's individual training has the advantage of increasing sexual vigor. This physiological invigoration occurs in two ways: as a general stimulation of the sexual glands and as a means of reinforcing the restraining power of the vaginal orifice where specific contractions are done. Such training in control can eventually result in a stage where the vaginal contraction can actually stop male ejaculation.

Beyond the now and then misleading interpretation of orgiastic deviations, the secret practice of the five "M"s actually culminates in a unique spiritual union. From a purely socioaesthetic point of view, it symbolizes tentatively the most beautiful moment in human relationship. In the Tantric world, however, such sexual union is not completely real. When either or both the playmates are successful in carrying out that sacred act, which presupposes the power to visualize and be intensively involved in *japa,* the sensuous realm is fully transcended, and thus allows an all-absorbing union with the beloved one, the *devatā* (see plate 19).

The following examples are but a glimpse of specific practices, orally instructed by a teacher supposed to be both competent and experienced, to qualified individuals who are fairly established in the Haṭha Yoga practice and have already achieved a high degree of control over their mental and bodily functions:

Individual training consists of special Haṭha Yoga techniques including anal contractions (Aśvinī Mudrā), Anal Lock (Mūla Bandha), movements with Anal Lock, vaginal contractions (Bhaga Śankaṣkriyā) along with pelvic retractions (Uḍḍīyāna Bandha), and drawing up in combination with Anal Lock; Penile Lock (Linga Śankaṣkriyā) and drawing up the penis with Anal Lock and pelvic Uḍḍīyāna; assuming Siddhāsana (Accomplished Posture) with Anal Lock, pelvic Uḍḍīyāna, diaphragmatic retractions, breath suspension (*kumbhaka*) with Chin Lock (Jālandhara Bandha) and Palatine Lock (Khecarī Mudrā). Modified Yoni Mudrā for both, while embracing and kissing each other in motionless coitus.

Practicing together, every evening, four or five hours before dinner, for a period of time up to three months. A quiet and nicely scented room with candlelight makes an appropriate stage setting for Lata Sādhana, the Tantric practice done by a couple. Sitting on cushions naked, at a distance from one another to escape body smell interference, with eyes closed and silent, is another requisite for the couple's parallel effort to ignore each other and commence the process with a preliminary exercise aimed at achieving relaxation of the body and mental calmness. This is followed by a steady one-hour practice of Sahita Prāṇāyāma, Alternate-Nostril Breath Control with Breath Suspension, *mūla japa,* and prayer.

Full chastity by sharing the same bed for sleep (occasionally changing sides) for a period of three months, naked and with no bodily contact.

Prolonged sexual intercourse (up to three hours), without allowing any seminal loss or with a single ejaculation, while the yogini may either fully contain orgasmic pressure or allow the release of several consecutive orgasms.

In a sublimated physical union, which is at the same time sensual and transcends the sensual, the two adepts aspire to unite themselves with their respective divinities. In the woman, the yogi will achieve union with the Goddess (Śakti); in the man, the yogini will realize the nature of the Lord (Śiva). The couple will thus symbolize the final Tantric immersion of any duality in Parama Śiva, the Supreme Being.

9
Ṣaṭ Karman–Purifications

In any belief, Gnostic or religious, purity is often a central and inseparable topic. Unrelated to the hypocrisy of conformism, it is a real *vade mecum* for any sincerely religious person, in the broadest sense of the term. It is in fact the virtue par excellence, which particularly makes it possible to realize in any spiritual search the truth stated by Saint Paul according to whom "all is pure for he who is pure."

Internal Purifications

From time immemorial, yogic literature has affirmed the importance of internal purifications (*śodhana*) as an essential condition for health, strength, development, and longevity. Inherent in the traditional practice of Haṭha Yoga, it is an established fact that these exercises assist greatly in energizing the whole organism.

A person on the path of Yoga is extremely conscious of the influence of *tamas,* the inertia that surrounds and inhabits us, which is both ignorance and impurity, whereas the yogi is naturally oriented toward lucidity, power, and mastery, toward an ideal of transcendence. The guru—by definition the dispeller of ignorance—teaches the aspirant how to recognize the many obstacles on the spiritual way, as well as the means to surmount them.

The yogi (or the yogini) can accept purifications from the outset, well knowing the importance of this jewel—purity—which, once fully established, will allow them to achieve the ideal, the emergence of a body similar to that of the gods (*deva deha*). Just as is implied by the Greek term *καθαρὸς,* which assimilates cleanliness and purity, for the practitioner of Yoga, cleanliness is inseparable from the state of purity that is aspired to and cherished. The purifying act provides structure to life, will on occasions become a ritual, and will inspire the yogi's quest for purity. The regular and prolonged practice of these purifications often has the spontaneous effect of awakening another need, that of making spiritual offerings. In the language of the poet: "Like the translucent morning dew, the purified soul reflects the light of the Creator."

Regrettably, the potential wealth of purifications in Yoga is somewhat ignored in our world, a world dedicated to curing diseases, well-being, and communication. However, no other school of thought can enrich the conception of hygiene as can Haṭha Yoga, which is a nurturing ground for cleanliness and purity. None of these purifications is mentioned in the Upaniṣads; they are found, however, in the Tantric literature dealing with Haṭha Yoga. Originating in the Tantric text *Aghamarṣana,* four methods of internal purification have evolved over time: the fivefold method of Bhairavi, the sixfold and eightfold methods of Śiva (*aṣṭa karman*), and the sixfold method of Gheranda.

These purifications deal on the one hand with the deep internal impurities of the organism, which require the application of Bhūta Śuddhi* and *prāṇāyāma;* they also concern the cleanliness of the tissues and organs of elimination, respectively.

To practice these various methods of internal cleansing, yogic students need first to follow the guru's directions and indispensable supervision. However, to truly master these techniques, they must also mobilize their own faculties, their determination and will, and apply them to the

***Bhūta Śuddhi* literally means the "cleaning of the (*mahā*)*bhūtas*." The term has different connotations depending on the yogic discipline concerned. In the Haṭha Yoga context it is best understood as an advanced purifying process that involves breath control with or without mantras. It is an important mental process that aims at eliminating all thought as it reproduces, virtually, the awakening of the Kuṇḍalinī, which is a very real experience.

control of the mind and muscles. A minimum of external means, such as the simple tongue scraper, will be enough, and air and water will achieve, for instance, the objective of nasopharyngeal cleaning.

Many criteria nourish the yogic ideal of purity. Yogis and yoginis do not conceive of their spiritual life only in terms of overall well-being, though this is an honorable ambition in itself. They know that beyond this they must have self-mastery in all the other phases of life. Yogis and yoginis are in fact comparable to warriors who have to fight on multiple fronts.

Included among their many objectives, with a concern for self-control underlying all, are enduring vitality, reduction of food wastes in the organism, body symmetry, and beauty and grace; in addition, they nurture the ambition of a clean and fragrant body, and effectiveness in action and thought. They seek energy and strength, endurance and serenity, and also the feeling of emotional fulfillment.

Of the four principal methods of internal purification, we will consider that of the yogi Gheranda, the most complete version. As its name indicates, *ṣaṭ karman* includes six acts:

1. **Dhautī:** cleansing, using air and water, of the digestive tract, stomach, oral cavity, and ears
2. **Vasti:** intestinal cleansing with air and water, which includes in particular Vāri Sāra and its easier variant Śaṇkprakṣalana
3. **Neti** (Nasal Cleansing): cleans the nasal cavities and upper section of the throat using water and cotton yarn
4. **Naulī** or **Laulikī** (Straight Muscle Exercise): fast gyratory movements of the rectus abdominis
5. **Trātaka** (Gazing): exercise involving visually focusing on an object to the point of shedding tears
6. **Kapālabhātī:** various nasopharyngeal techniques; in accordance with the method of Śivaism, the exercise of Kapālabhātī consists, in the practical teaching of Sri S. S. Goswami, of vigorous diaphragmatic hyperventilation

Neti is an easy form of cleaning renowned for preventing colds and stimulating the nervous system of the eye. Yogis usually rely on no mechanical aid, neti pot or the like, when practicing this exercise, which consists of sucking up one glass of lukewarm, salty water through the nostrils and immediately throwing it out through the mouth. In the next phase, cold water is retained in the mouth and immediately rejected through the nostrils.

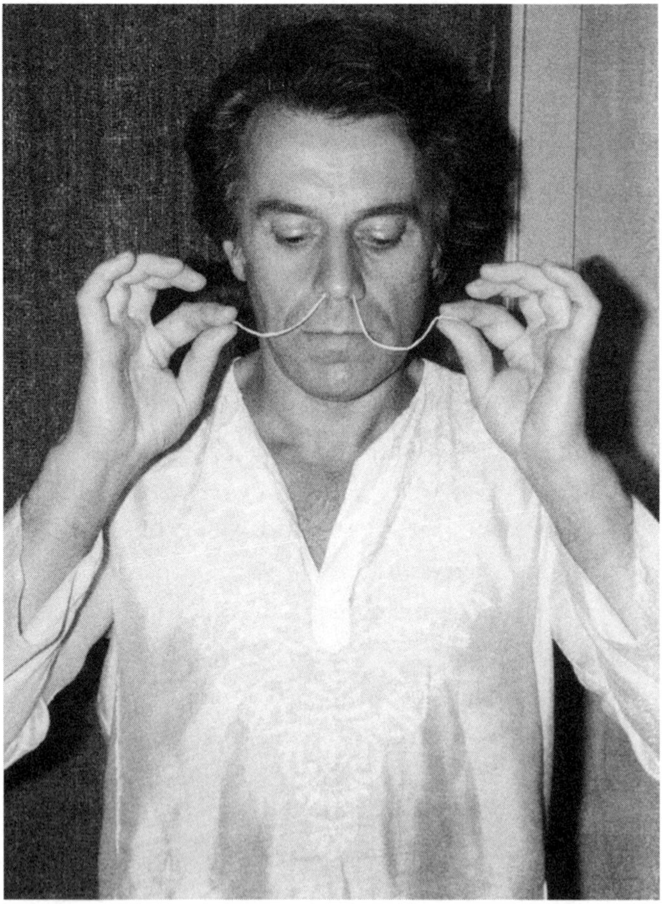

Fig. 9.1. Sūtra Neti (Nasal Thread-Cleansing)

Sūtra Neti (Nasal Thread-Cleansing) consists of introducing a thoroughly boiled cotton thread into one nostril and expelling it via the mouth, then repeating with the other nostril. In the next and final phase, the thread is passed from one nostril into the other, as shown in the figure below, first in one direction, then the other.

The multiform control of the rectus abdominis and its two adjacent semilunar lines, which is practiced in Naulī or Laulikī (Straight Muscle Exercise) is a typical yogic discovery. Besides developing the mental power to control—mostly by way of visualization, given that the exercise requires no significant muscular effort—the isolation of the central abdominal muscle illustrates clearly the pragmatic concerns to be found in the philosophy of Haṭha Yoga. The original yogic purpose of Naulī is to provide a natural means for auto-lavage (with no mechanical aid), which is possible when the anal muscles are fully relaxed.

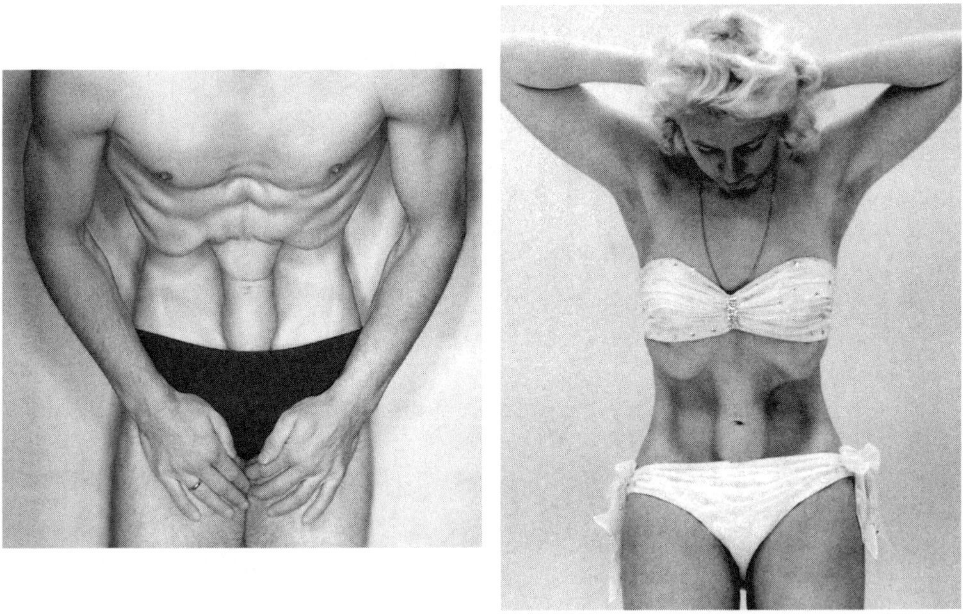

Fig. 9.2. Naulī or Laulikī (Straight Muscle Exercise), control of the rectus abdominis

Only after having regularly practiced the six purifications will the yogi be able to begin the practice of *prāṇāyāma* (described in the next chapter), which is designed to eradicate deep internal impurities. Briefly let us note the method of Nāḍī Suddhi, an important component of the higher stages of the practice of *prāṇāyāma*. Nāḍī Śuddhi consists of removing any obstacle in the subtle intermediate sphere between the body and mind (*nāḍī cakra*), with the correct operation of the kinetic

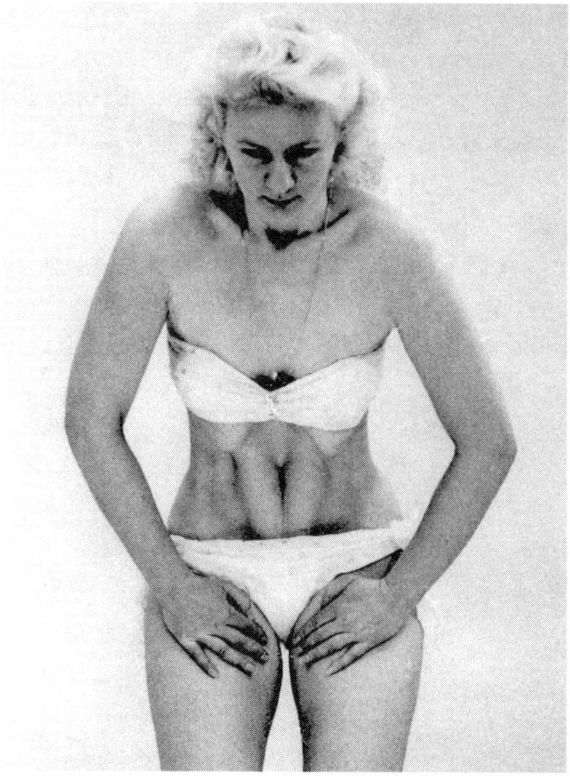

Fig. 9.3. Separate isolation of the abdominal recti

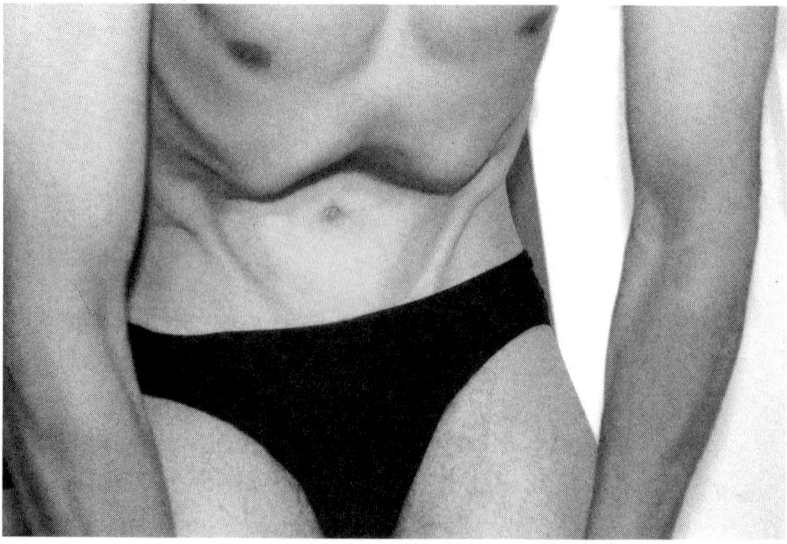

Fig. 9.4. Advanced abdominal control unveiling the lineae semilunares

forces (*vāyu*) of *prāṇa*—in particular two principal forces, one solar, *idā,* the other lunar, *pingalā,* as well as the stabilizing force, *suṣumnā,* which balances them in perfect harmony.

Advanced Exercises of Control

The advanced exercises of control involve the following procedures:

Vamana Dhautī (Gastric Auto-Lavage): In this process of self-cleansing of the stomach, the pupil drinks water and then vomits it, naturally, without external assistance. This method allows the washing of the stomach and reinforces the muscles involved.

Jala Vasti (Colonic Auto-Lavage): In this process of self-cleansing of the large intestine, the pupil draws up water through the rectum without mechanical assistance in order to clean the colon.

Śuṣka Vasti (Colonic Auto-Air Bath): This is atmospheric self-cleansing, in which the student draws in air through the rectum without mechanical assistance. The procedure is also used in *prāṇāyāma.*

Vāri Sāra (Alimentary Canal Auto-Lavage): In this process of self-cleansing of the digestive tract, the student drinks water, makes it pass from the stomach to the small intestine, then through the large intestine, finally expelling it via the anus, thus discharging all the fecal contents with it. This method is particularly effective for cleansing, without external assistance, the entire digestive tract.

Śankprakṣalana (Auto-Lavage of the Alimentary Canal): As effective but easier to perform than Vāri Sāra, this variation of self-cleansing of the digestive tract is carried out by drinking water in alternation with four movements.

Vāta Sāra (Alimentary Canal Auto-Air Bath): In this atmospheric self-cleansing of the digestive tract, the pupil swallows air, makes it pass from the stomach to the small intestine, then to the large intestine, finally ejecting it via the anus without mechanical assistance. This procedure is mainly used in advanced *prāṇāyāma.*

Vajrolī Mudrā: This is the most difficult of control achievements in Haṭha Yoga (see chapters 7 and 8 for details relating to this practice).

10
Prāṇāyāma—Respiratory Control

Haṭha Yoga teaches us that, in addition to the maintenance of a posture (*āsana*) in perfect immobility, the other condition required to reach deep mental concentration is the control of breathing (*prāṇāyāma*).

Prāṇa

The study of the fourth part of Haṭha Yoga supposes a high level of interest, as much for the practitioner as for the reader who is curious about the nature of *prāṇa* or the practice of *prāṇāyāma*. The term *prāṇa* signifies an idea with no equivalent in the Western world. It refers to the original principle of an energetic power inherent in any cosmic manifestation—a holistic, immanent energy that creates life itself, matter, and the world of the mind. In the following account, *prāṇa* will be presented only as this vital principle that underlies human life, a kinetic principle that the yogi uses in an important stage of spiritual research. To facilitate comprehension of the term, it can be simply translated as "vital force."

Certain authors, probably inspired by the New Age movement, have wanted to make connections between mysticism (to which Yoga is often related) and research on the part of the scientific community, in particular in physics. However, the thesis of a primordial principle of universal energy does not feature among the concerns of the scientific community, whose spheres of interest are at the level of what is tangible, measurable, quantifiable, rational, and utilitarian. Though it is relatively easy to measure the pranic force expressed at the respiratory level, along with physiological and neurological modifications, it is more difficult to apprehend the nature of the operation of this pervasive primordial power, *prāṇa*. It is no less difficult to describe in rational terms the higher state of consciousnesses reached by yogis in *samyama,* which results specifically from the control of this same *prāṇa*.

The scientific validity of the Hindu conception of *prāṇa* cannot be found in any research results from the physical sciences nor in explanations coming from science in general, whose truths fluctuate according to whatever doctrine is in fashion. Obviously, scientific theories are subject to the passage of time, contrary to their object of study, which generally remains unchanged. In the Hindu conception, the physical sphere is at the lowest level of an extremely complex scale. Evolution here is the result of a timeless projection of the Supreme Consciousness, which itself generates a causality that, in turn, gives rise to an omnipresent subtle vital sphere, *prāṇa*. In a person, *prāṇa vāyu* is the bridge reaching toward the mind, which is nothing less than the dominant part of our being. *Prāṇa* takes form and substance in a materiality where the individual, like a timeless Diogenes, uses the weak lantern of intellect and intuition to seek a Truth that is forever out of reach.

Prāṇa is the global power that becomes altered when in contact with *puruṇa,* the basic principle of consciousness and *prakṛiti* (φύση or nature), the potential of the cosmos and all the phenomena, including the mind. The developments and multiple manifestations of *prāṇa* give access to an intermediate world, the vital world (*nāḍī cakra*), which is the constantly active sphere connecting the physical and mental realms, or, in conventional language, the body and soul.

While *prāṇa* infuses life into all organic matter, *prāṇāyāma* allows the return to the latent state of *prāṇa*. In a pranic state, which is by nature supramental, the body is inanimate but enlightened by a massive interior consciousness (*ghana prajña*). From the yogic point of view, this state contradicts the scientific epistemological assumption according to which the mind is ultimately only a product of complex cerebral activities.

Nāḍīs and *Vāyus*

The sacred writings of the Vedas and of Tantric literature mention the sphere of *nāḍīs,* the *nāḍī cakra.* Derived from the Sanskrit word *nāda,* this term indicates "that which radiates," "the kinetic," or "that which has to do with movement." Whether physical or subtle (in which case the term *yogannāḍī* is used), the Tantras teach that the *nāḍīs* are innumerable. In Yoga, this aspect allows the reconnection of the subtle world to the sensory world.

The subtle body of a person is composed of three principal *nāḍīs.* The first, *idā,* appears in lunar form (*candra*) and the second, *pingalā,* symbolizes the sun (*sūrya*). These two subtle currents assume the passage of the vital current, which passes through the nostrils from atmospheric air. Usually inactive, the third, *suṣumnā,* plays an important role in the passage of Kuṇḍalinī (the Grand Spiritual Potential of Consciousness) through the different *cakras* (energy centers). Inseparable from the *nāḍīs* are the *vāyus* (also called *prāṇa vāyus*), the kinetic manifestation of the pranic force. Of the ten *vāyus,* five assume an essential role in the expression of *prāṇa's* state of perpetual motion: *prāṇa, apāna, samāna, udāna,* and *vyāna.* To summarize Sri S. S. Goswami's technical interpretation of these subtle elements, the *nāḍīs* are the pranic expression of radiating lines, inseparable from the movements (*vāyus*) of *prāṇa.*

Strictly from the point of view of Haṭha Yoga, breathing is much more than the expression of our vitality or the movement of the organs, which are our lungs, heart, and all the muscles involved in the vital processes. For the yogi, breathing is the physiological expression of a vital kinetic current (*prāṇa vāyu*), an aerobic manifestation closely related to the mental life, which primarily expresses an orientation that is characteristic of awareness of the outside, together with a spontaneous inward movement.

Practice of the Discipline

While *prāṇa* is effectively mentioned in the Vedic literature, the word *prāṇāyāma,* on the other hand, does not appear there. Patañjali introduced the Brāhmaṇic term into the discipline of Haṭha Yoga. According to his *Yoga Sūtras,* the practice of *prāṇāyāma* allows the elimination of that which obstructs the light of the vital body (II.52) and prepares the adept for mental concentration (II.53). Practitioners of *prāṇāyāma* have long observed the interaction of the mind and breathing and been aware of the influence of this natural phenomenon on the flow of the mind. In this way, they have shown its positive effects on the immune system, physical development, and the strength of the whole organism.

The discipline of *prāṇāyāma* is divided into two principal categories: respiratory control (or mastery of the breath) and concentration. In Haṭha Yoga, *prāṇāyāma* is done in association with dynamic *āsanas* and *cāraṇā*. The practice of voluntary breath control is usually done in crossed-leg sitting posture. To be efficient, the practice should be undertaken with an empty stomach and a quiet, well-controlled mind. The surroundings should be silent and clean. If the practice is just for the purpose of wellness, it should be done outdoors.

The exercises of voluntary breathing are broken down into three phases: hyperventilation, hypoventilation, and retention or suspension of the breath (or apnea). Voluntary hyperventilation is divided into two forms: it can be diaphragmatic (Kapālabhātī) or thoracic (Bhastrikā). Practiced regularly in the teaching of the Goswami Yoga Institute, these respiratory exercises in particular have permitted the reconsideration of maximal hyperventilation previously expressed in handbooks on the physiology of the human lung. Until quite recently it was thought that voluntary hyperventilation could not exceed 100 breaths per minute. However, the pupils of the Goswami Institute have reached voluntary frequencies of hyperventilation much higher than this limit. The hyperventilation of *prāṇāyāma* allows one to go from 60 to 120 breaths per minute, finally attaining a standard of 240 breaths. Certain established students of Sri Goswami exhibited periods of hyperventilation exceeding 300 breaths per minute! Another teaching, drawn from the practice of Kapālabhātī

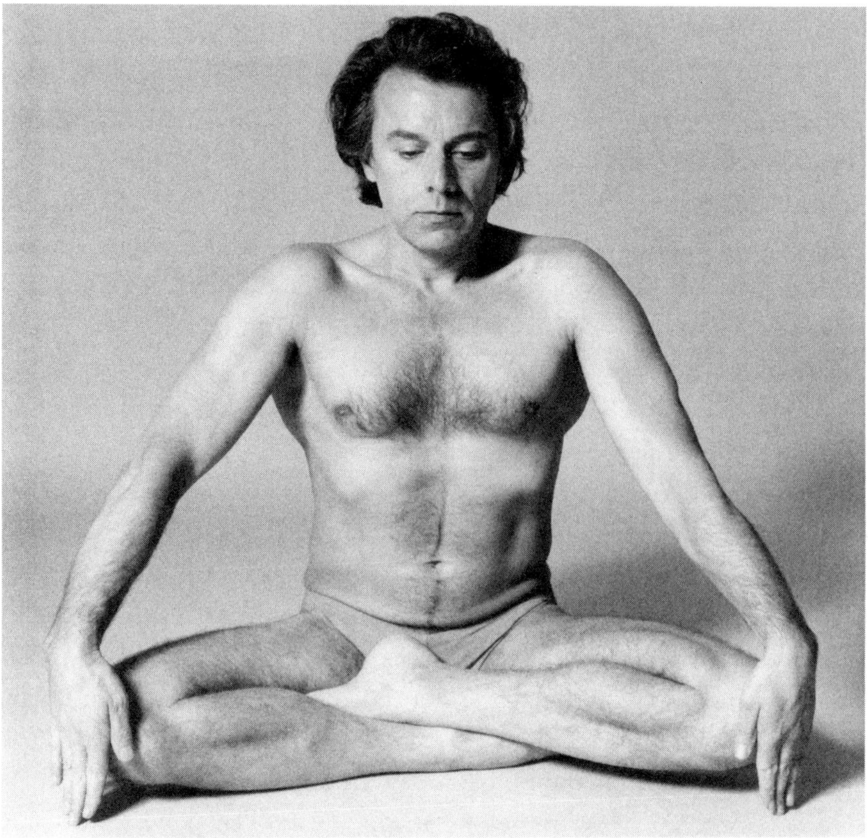

Fig. 10.1. *Prāṇāyāma* generally starts with a prolonged period of either abdominal (Kapālabhātī) or thoracic (Bhastrikā) hyperventilation, soon followed by long-slow breathing exercises, with or without breath suspension. Advanced breath control leads to automatic apnea and modified consciousness. In exceptional cases, it may induce body levitation.

and Bhastrikā, is the fact that regular and prolonged exercise makes it possible to avoid the risk of acidosis, even when yogic hyperventilation is maintained without interruption during an hour or more.*

The individual's natural phases of breathing are methodically

*C. Frostell, J. N. Pande, and G. Hedenstierna, "Effects of High-Frequency Breathing on Pulmonary Ventilation and Gas Exchange," *Journal of Applied Physiology* 55, no. 6 (December 1): 1983.

modulated by the prolongation, reduction, or cessation of inhalation or exhalation. The terms for these three components of the respiratory exercises—*pūraka* (controlled inhalation), *recaka* (controlled exhalation), and *kumbhaka* (controlled retention or suspension)—appear in the Upaniṣads, Tantras, and Purāṇas, as well as in modern yogic terminology.

Of these three phases of respiratory control, the retention of the breath is regarded as most important because it particularly promotes the faculty of concentration. However, when a man or woman suffers from psychosomatic imbalance, the mind is functioning on a more subtle level than that of the body. It is then impossible to prolong the retention of the breath in a truly beneficial way for the practice of mental concentration. To try and retain the breath by a physical effort at this point scarcely makes sense, except for the development of willpower.

The control of the breath is done in stages. Only the accomplished practitioner in the discipline of *prāṇāyāma* will be able to progress toward perfection, while at the same time not neglecting the body. It is possible to affect the level of mental tranquility and physical immobility by determining the frequency and depth of breathing. The maintenance of a motionless and stable body for a long period makes it possible to considerably decrease the frequency as well as the amplitude of breathing. Gradually, this exercise becomes easy for the practitioner insofar as the mind becomes increasingly calm and concentration deeper. At a certain level of development, the practitioner's breathing will become barely perceptible: breathing of the *hamsa* type, which precedes the total and spontaneous suspension of the breath (*kevala kumbhaka*). It is also one of the yogi's aims to awaken the Kuṇḍalinī using *prāṇāyāma*.

From the above, it emerges that the state that best suits mental concentration is in direct opposition to any state that favors movement. In addition, let us underline that beyond the goals and specific results of *prāṇāyāma,* the practice of this discipline produces effects of well-being that are far from negligible. They seem to us worthy of mention.

- First of all, the regular practice of *prāṇāyāma* helps the practitioner to reinforce and gain greater mastery of all the physical elements involved: muscles, lungs, heart, arteries, and nervous system. Energy is increased and ventilation improved.

Moreover, it permits awareness of the benefits arising from complete breathing, such as a better control of the senses and increased tone of the organs—in particular, peristalsis, those wave-like alternate contraction and relaxation movements in the alimentary canal that progressively push forward its contents.

Combined with other exercises like *āsanas,* purifications, and a suitable diet, the regular practice of *prāṇāyāma* promotes good health and physical performance.

Another advantage of a regular practice of *prāṇāyāma* is to make it possible for the individual to experience privileged moments, sublime impulses, elevation of the soul, strokes of genius, or waves of spiritual immersion. However, to be complete, the practice of higher *prāṇāyāma* supposes sexual control, or *brahmacarya,* lest the practitioner's health is put at risk.

In short, the discipline of *prāṇāyāma* makes the yogi virtuous—in the etymological sense of the Latin term *virtus,* a valorous person who is aware of his or her strength.

The historical evolution of this technique saw the development of many versions of the ancient discipline of *prāṇāyāma*. On a higher level, the advanced yogi, subjected to a strict milk diet, will practice the control of *prāṇa* over periods ranging from nine to twelve hours per day. It is at the end of the final phase of Sahita Prāṇāyāma, characterized by the spontaneous cessation of breathing (*kevala kumbhaka*), that the rare antigravitational phenomenon of levitation occurs.

When it published the picture shown in fig. 10.2 *The Illustrated London News* reported:

> The levitation lasted for about 10 minutes including 5 minutes for the yogi to come down from the top position to the ground. On one shot at the initial stage, the yogi's face appears to be quite normal. However, during the raising of the body clear signs of fatigue appear, the turban falls down, the hand on the stick appears more

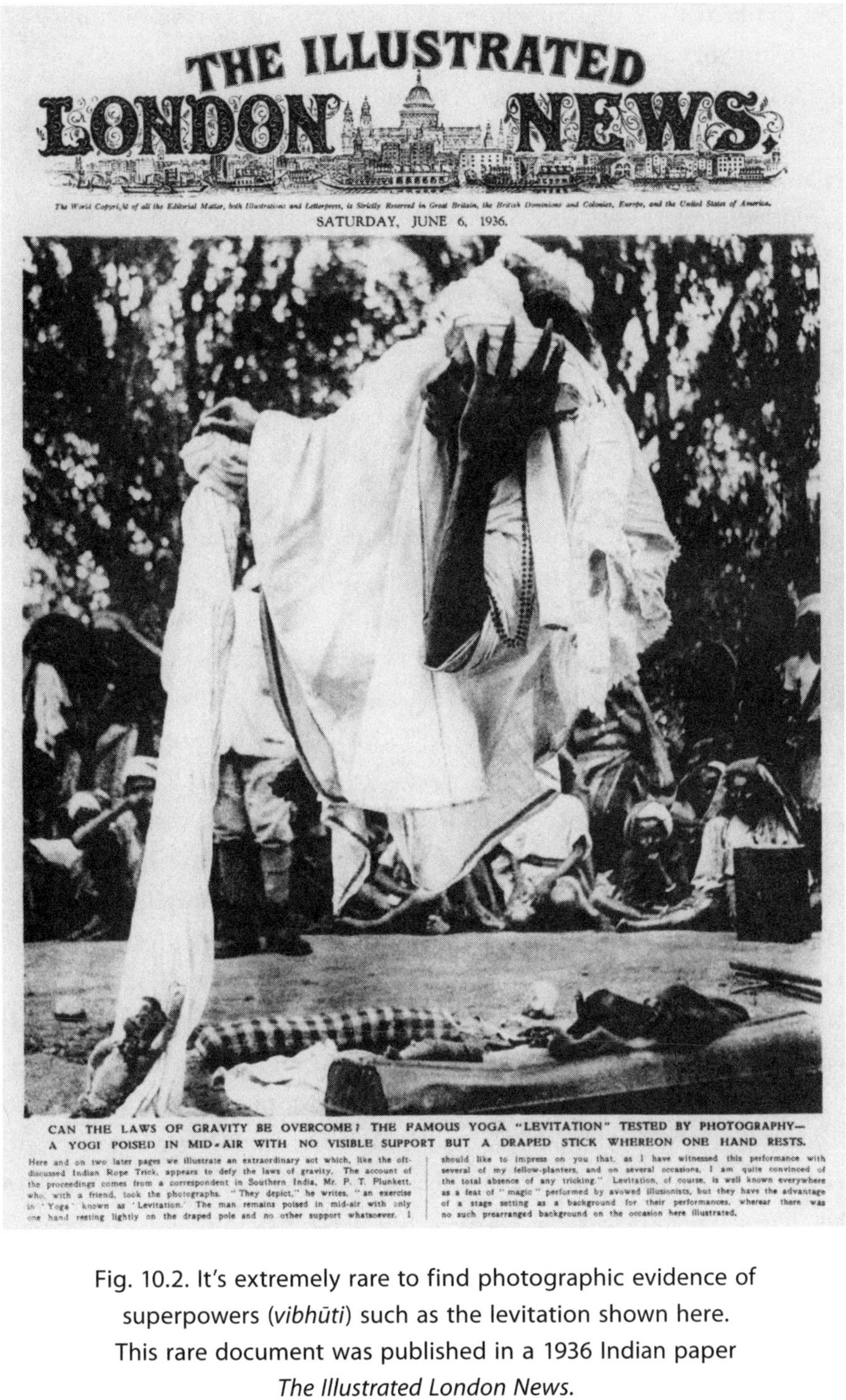

THE ILLUSTRATED LONDON NEWS,

The World Copyright of all the Editorial Matter, both Illustrations and Letterpress, is Strictly Reserved in Great Britain, the British Dominions and Colonies, Europe, and the United States of America.

SATURDAY, JUNE 6, 1936.

CAN THE LAWS OF GRAVITY BE OVERCOME? THE FAMOUS YOGA "LEVITATION" TESTED BY PHOTOGRAPHY—A YOGI POISED IN MID-AIR WITH NO VISIBLE SUPPORT BUT A DRAPED STICK WHEREON ONE HAND RESTS.

Here and on two later pages we illustrate an extraordinary act which, like the oft-discussed Indian Rope Trick, appears to defy the laws of gravity. The account of the proceedings comes from a correspondent in Southern India, Mr. P. T. Plunkett, who, with a friend, took the photographs. "They depict," he writes, "an exercise in 'Yoga' known as 'Levitation.' The man remains poised in mid-air with only one hand resting lightly on the draped pole and no other support whatsoever. I should like to impress on you that, as I have witnessed this performance with several of my fellow-planters, and on several occasions, I am quite convinced of the total absence of any tricking." Levitation, of course, is well known everywhere as a feat of "magic" performed by avowed illusionists, but they have the advantage of a stage setting as a background for their performances, wherear there was no such prearranged background on the occasion here illustrated.

Fig. 10.2. It's extremely rare to find photographic evidence of superpowers (*vibhūti*) such as the levitation shown here. This rare document was published in a 1936 Indian paper *The Illustrated London News.*

contracted and the countenance shows signs of inner tension culminating in an expression of exhaustion when reaching the ground. By passing a stick above, underneath and around the yogi's body, the British observer of this feat of superhuman powers checked that the performance was actually no fake, and ensured that there was no other support than the stick on which the yogi's hand was resting.

Nāḍī Śuddhi

The purification of the body is closely related to Nāḍī Śuddhi, an important subdiscipline of Haṭha Yoga. With this method, the body is completely purified and the slowest of its vibrations is modified, so that they are able to mix with the subtlest mental vibrations. From the point of view of the mind, it becomes calmer, more focused, and joyful, with subtler vibrations and elevated thoughts. Purified, the body no longer has a cumbersome influence on the mind. Through Nāḍī Śuddhi the body is cleaned, revitalized, and rebalanced. It becomes healthier and lighter, and it releases a pleasant fragrance.

Nāḍī Śuddhi includes Samanu (which, in *prāṇāyāma,* is referred to as Nāḍī Śuddhi Prāṇāyāma) and Nirmanu or acts of body purification, commonly called *ṣaṭ karman* (six acts). The method known as Nāḍī Śuddhi Prāṇāyāma consists of a process of internal muscular contraction intended to allow prolongation of the apnea. This contraction is caused by Jālandhara Bandha (Chin Lock), Uḍḍīyāna Bandha (Abdominal Retraction), and Mūla Bandha (Anal Lock). The method insists on these three simultaneous contractions being performed maximally. To reinforce the first contraction, two special exercises are envisaged: Meru Cālana (Throat Exercise) and Mani Cālana (Trunk and Throat Exercise). It should be also noted that the pressure exerted on the abdominal cavity during Uḍḍīyāna and Mūla Bandha will not give the required effect if the intestine is not perfectly clean. This is the very raison d'être of the different purifying exercises prescribed by yogis, detailed in the previous chapter, "*Ṣaṭ Karman*—Purifications."

The advanced technique of Khecarī Mudrā makes it possible to obtain an internal pressure capable of facilitating the retention of breath. Rare are the practitioners who will use this difficult exercise, which requires intense training under the supervision of a qualified teacher. The method, which supposes many preliminary manipulations, consists of an introversion of the tongue that, folded up on itself, must penetrate toward the back of the oral cavity until it covers the glottis. The point of the folded tongue blocks the respiratory tracts and creates a degree of internal pressure. Jālandhara Bandha and Mūla Bandha are parts of the practice of Khecarī. Practiced in an inverted posture, this method is then called Viparītakaraṇī Mudrā.

Svara Yoga

Svara Yoga, a little known variation of *prāṇāyāma,* is an ancient, special discipline based primarily on the principles of *prānāyāmic* control of the *prāṇa* and *nāḍīs,* the kinetic lines of the vital force. The pragmatism of Svara Yoga is expressed in the control over the relation that exists between breath and psyche. It has been adopted by certain yogis for whom life is not measured in terms of days and years, but by the rhythm of their own breathing. The intensity of the passage of air through our nostrils varies during normal breathing. The air goes through our nostrils in an alternating process, according to an infradian biological cycle (a period longer than twenty-four hours) that differs appreciably from the circadian one, which is to say it is considerably less than a day. In India, nasal respiratory alternation is an age-old recognized physiological phenomenon.

The practitioner of Svara Yoga excels in the knowledge of the complex phenomenon of *prāṇa* and of the *nāḍīs.* Thanks to the study, observations, and experiments of yogic predecessors who have investigated the respiratory cycle, practitioners can in turn discover the subtle changes that occur in their organism, in particular the correlation that exists between breathing and the mind. They will also learn, with the assistance of appropriate techniques, how to modify the alternation of their breathing at will and at their own pace.

When the breath is more pronounced on the right side, it is the influence of *pingalā,* a "solar" energetic principle, which is represented symbolically by the god-awareness Śiva. More marked breathing on the left side is "lunar," which is a tendency of the *idā nāḍī,* represented by the power of Śakti. The first predominance denotes dynamism and extraversion, while the second expresses its opposite, introspection and quietude.

This empirical knowledge symbolically reveals the characteristic inherent dualism* of the human condition. By subtly observing their breath, yogis can determine their choice of action in the immediate future and the perfect moment for each one of their actions, such as meals, rest, travel, in short all the activities of life, sacred or social.

It is at the heart of this practice, beyond the contingencies of a life of constraints, that the yogi will endeavor to equalize the pranic *idā* and *pingalā* currents into a perfect balance, in the third main *nāḍī*—*suṣumnā*. It is precisely this union of binary energies, which corresponds to the fusion of the forces *ha* and *ṭha,* that is peculiar to the discipline of Haṭha Yoga. The retraction of the mind from the object of the senses, *pratyāhāra,* which precedes profound mental concentration, occurs at the end of *prāṇāyāma*.

*Yogic discoveries and their variations are probably not unrelated to the current differing interpretations concerning the two brain hemispheres.

11
Pratyāhāra–Control of the Senses

For the rishi, each of us is only a wave in a vast ocean, a limited manifestation of an immanent, eternal, immeasurable Power-Reality that is consequently imperceptible by ordinary consciousness. Spiritually motivated and pragmatic, the doctrine of Yoga is trivalent—vision, method, and realization all at the same time. It assumes the union of self, by immersion of one's identity, with an impenetrable Reality. Without denying its purpose as a pathway for the person of action, Yoga has revealed, and today still teaches, the secret of inaction within a continual movement of the mind.

While it is relatively easy to control the body, the control of the mind is decidedly more difficult. The mind is constantly on the watch for *vṛittis*—sensory images, feelings, and emotions, which unceasingly monopolize the waking state. At times, however, we withdraw, quite unconsciously, our attention from the objects that surround us, for example when we are deeply absorbed in an activity, a problem, or during a telephone conversation.

In the waking state, we are directly conscious of the sensory world through our five senses—hearing, sight, smell, taste, and touch—and the organs corresponding to these faculties of perception. With our cognitive senses, we experience the thousands of impressions, feelings, and emotions that relentlessly solicit our attention. These various sensory impressions are first conveyed by an electrochemical biological process, then they are transformed automatically into precise mental images, and finally selected and synthesized on the basis of genetic, cultural, or aesthetic criteria, which are unique to the individual. Thus, for a very brief moment we retain a particular object in the objective field of our consciousness, which will be replaced at once by another object of our choice.

However, according to the doctrine of Yoga, the control of the mind makes it effectively possible to cut the bond that connects the senses to the external objects of the sensory world. This is precisely the meaning of the root *hri* of the Sanskrit word *pratyāhāra:* "to move away"; in other words, to keep the senses away from their object and thus prevent the formation of new sensory images within a mental vacuum. This method implies mental immersion, withdrawal within (into) the mind, which temporarily separates a person from the external world.

Unlike during sleep—where, in particular, the organs of hearing, smell, and touch (and sometimes even sight, in the case of people who sleep with half-opened eyes) are potentially receptive to the perception of sensory objects—in *pratyāhāra,* the yogi does not sleep but is perfectly awake and is sometimes even in an intense state of awareness.

This fifth discipline of the eightfold path of Yoga, *pratyāhāra,* does not appear in the Vedic Samhītās or in the Brāhmaṇas. The process is mentioned in several Upaniṣads, sometimes in allegorical form, for example when Goraksha Paddhati reminds the yogi that he must withdraw his senses into himself, following the example of the tortoise, which folds up its limbs inside its carapace. But references in the Upaniṣads also can be technical, as in their advice to associate *pratyāhāra* with the practice of *kumbhaka* (apnea) (*Yogatattvopaniṣad* 69) or with mental concentration, in particular on eighteen vital centers of the body (*Triśikhibrāmanopaniṣad* 2.129–130 and *Śāṇḍilya,* 1.8.1–2.).

The introspective method of *pratyāhāra* is conveyed to us in a pithy presentation of two of Patañjali's sutras, which designate a mind emptied of the external object of the senses, a state where consciousness withdraws from the external world that unceasingly solicits it.

The special feature of the process of *pratyāhāra* is that it has no goal other than the suspension of the external flood of mental images, abandoning to mental concentration the task of surmounting the obstacle created by all the other images, memorized or projected in anticipation. The practitioner of Haṭha Yoga will remember that the success of this discipline—an unavoidable path for climbing the steps of *samyama* (the various phases of mental concentration)—is closely related to the preliminary exercises, that is, the practice of the ten ethical rules of *yama* and *niyama,* as well as control of the body using *āsanas* and of the breath using *prāṇāyāma.*

12
Stages of Concentration

Thoughts can be groups of images that appear in the objective field (*citta*) of our consciousness. Generally the images forming a group are closely linked. A group can be simple and limited, or complex and extended. Thoughts, such as they appear to the ego (*aham*), are either simple images of the memory of our daily experiences or they form a constructive idea, even a brilliant one.

The level of our mental life is determined by the type of thought that dominates it. At lower mental stages, thought can express a blindness in which darkness, indolence, and lack of attention, intelligence, or comprehension are its main features. In an agitated state, thoughts are dominated by wishes, desires, greed, or excesses. On the other hand, in a mind intensely "monofocal," that is to say concentrating on only one object, thoughts are sharp, constructive, noble, and elevated. In reality, thoughts are an image of a person's self.

A thought is not just something that comes and goes. Our thoughts not only influence the mind. They deeply mark the brain, the nervous system, the internal organs, and the whole body. Destructive thought makes us less controlled, more petty, egoistic, weak, and physically imperfect. On the other hand, constructive thought develops creative energies, strength, health, and a broader perspective. Weak thoughts really do not encourage action; they are maintained only momentarily in the mind and then quickly disappear from it. Strong thoughts, on the contrary, promote action. Feeling can reinforce thought. The constructive or destructive character of a thought thus depends on the type of feeling that is associated with it.

Thought also has another aspect, which remains hidden from a normally functioning mind. On a level where everything is transmitted by the senses, there is no awareness unless it is in combination with certain vibrations. Moreover, we are only conscious of the grosser forms of vibrations. These forms are associated with the fast and uninterrupted formation of our consciousness based on the objects that give rise to the mental images of our awareness of the external world. We constantly spend our mental energy on rapid sequences in the field of our consciousness, instead of transforming it into a truly alive form or a stimulant for action, which is then recorded as a subliminal impression that, in the future, can be recalled at will. The only way of developing and controlling this hidden force is to try to move from a state of dispersion to a form of monofocal thought. This form is called *ekāgratā*. It is the mental exercise that consists of seizing and retaining a single image.

Experience shows that it is almost impossible to maintain at will a given mental image for a prolonged time. A new image pushes back the first one, and then another appears when the second disappears, and so on. Mental energy is dissipated without our realizing what is in fact happening. Yoga is the means of preventing this needless dissipation of energy in the form of *vṛittis* (the continual formation of consciousness derived from sensory objects) and to develop the faculty of maintaining a single image in the mind. It is here that true concentration begins. Yoga teaches us how to control the insane rush of our mind and to develop our faculty of concentration.

Dhāraṇā, *Dhyāna*, and *Samādhi*

It is customary to distinguish three stages of concentration, referred to by the terms *dhāraṇā, dhyāna,* and *samādhi.*

Dhāraṇā is the first stage, when an appropriate object is selected for the mind to concentrate upon. It is characteristic of the mind to manifest various sequential images, each of which is retained for only a brief moment. *Dhāraṇā* is the method in which the mind retains the selected image and recaptures it as soon as it escapes in order to continue to maintain it without allowing another image to take its place. *Dhāraṇā* is the process of intermittently establishing the same single image in the mind. This sequential image process can be compared with the falling of water, drop by drop, from a perforated vessel full of water.

When concentration deepens, it is possible to maintain only one focused image without it escaping from the mind. At this point, the drop-by-drop stream changes into a continuous flow. It can be compared to oil or honey running slowly out of the spout of a carafe. This focusing of the consciousness is called *dhyāna*.

With practice, focusing becomes increasingly complete until finally the selected object alone illuminates one's whole consciousness. Everything else disappears from the mind. The yogi is then only aware of the subjective aspect of consciousness. The state of the mind in which concentration is at its apogee is called *samādhi*. In *samādhi,* any conscious form of bodily activity disappears to the point of forgetting the body, which then becomes completely motionless. At this stage, the adept becomes aware of a separate existence of the body and acquires extrasensory perception.

This experience has two categories, supramaterial and immaterial. In the first category, there is the faculty of perceiving objects or events from the past, present, or future relating to the sensory world, without the intervention of the senses. In the second category, there is the perception of phenomena that cannot be reached normally by the senses. There then emerges a new world of colors and forms that, via various intermediate stages, leads to ultimate, completely sublimated suprasensory knowledge. On this level, various types of latent powers appear, whereas normally they could never be expressed.

Samprajñāta Samādhi

Samprajñāta samādhi comprises various levels. The first stage is called *vitarka samādhi*. This involves choosing an object of concentration, a pattern of a sensory kind, a product of the five senses. What appears to us as a homogeneous object is actually a combination of the mixed functions of five potential forces called *bhūtas.* When they are combined or are presented to our minds, they take a material form.

In *dhāraṇā,* as in *dhyāna,* the object of mental concentration is sensory and material. In *vitarka samādhi,* the object changes character: an individual *bhūta* can be isolated from a group and used as an object of concentration. Thus each *bhūta* can be individualized and "seen" in *samādhi.* By this method, an aspect of the object is revealed that is not part of its sensory form; it is a suprasensory realization of our material world. The objective aspect of our consciousness acquires a new perspective, the image of a *bhūta* that, by nature, is suprasensory.

Even deeper concentration brings about the stage called *vicāra samādhi,* in which it becomes possible to distinguish the subtlest form of *bhūtas,* the *tanmātras.* Our image of the material world is then completely transformed. Sensory perceptions or other knowledge of our material world depend on vibrations that influence the senses. Each vibration taken separately is so fast and refined that it cannot be recorded on the level of the senses. The senses react only when confronted with the grouping of a great number of such vibrations, and the result is our usual coarse sensory consciousness. Each one of these subtle movements separately produces subtle knowledge, inaccessible to our senses. When a more solid foundation is acquired in *samādhi,* it becomes possible to reach this subtler knowledge, which is *tanmātra,* or dematerialized object.

The third stage is called *ānanda samādhi.* What characterizes this stage is the revelation of the root of our conception of the material world, a phenomenon called *abhimāna.* Its function appears by the simple fact of the relation that exists between ego and non-ego. At the human stage, consciousness consists of the ego, the subject, an object, and their mutual relationship. The feeling of ego is the Self plus some other thing. This other thing appears when the Self functions under the influence of *rajas,* the dynamic *guna* principle of change, which presents itself as that which knows and acts. The Self becomes identified with this non-self. The Self linked to the non-self is *ahamkāra.* In *ānanda samādhi,* concentration is so deep that the faculties of knowledge and action are fully developed, depriving *abhimāna* of any power over them. It is at this stage that human beings may experience the highest form of happiness.

The last stage of *samprajñāta samādhi* is called *asmitā samādhi.* On our ordinary level, it is impossible to isolate the Self from the non-self, because we are aware of the ego only via *abhimāna.* When *abhimāna* is controlled during a very significant effort of concentration, the Self is isolated from the phenomenon of the non-self and appears as one "infinite" Self. Objective images disappear from consciousness and only the Self remains. Consciousness takes the form of a pure Self that is the Self in its totality. The ego, freed from *abhimāna,* becomes *mahat. Sattva,* the principle of consciousness, then prevails. In *asmitā samādhi,* its revelation is complete.

Asamprajñāta Samādhi

The apogee of mental concentration is called *asamprajñāta samādhi.* At this stage, the image of the object, like that of the ego (*mahat*), is completely erased from consciousness, which is then formed neither by the object nor even by the purified ego. "Knowledge," as we usually conceive it, comes from the Self without any intermediary. This is what it means to know oneself, in oneself and by oneself, without external assistance. The dualistic form of our existence reaches a stage in which an eternal and immutable principle reigns, beyond birth and death. Consciousness becomes pure consciousness. Released from the least spot of impurity, it becomes supraconsciousness, beyond the realm of human existence. This is known as the appearance of *puruṇa.* In yogic terms, this state is called *yogacittavṛitti nirodha.*

Such a state of consciousness should not be regarded as a form of mental degeneration, nor be compared with an extinguished mental life, synonymous with "living death." It is not a dark state of the human organism, nor a disastrous metamorphosis of the mind. On the contrary, it is a hidden face of human existence appearing at this stage of *samādhi,* which is in fact a total broadening of our limited existence, the elevation of awareness to the highest form that human consciousness can reach.* The body and mind function normally when the state of *samādhi* ceases, which proves that this state is not an abnormal one. The fact is that in this state, thinking gains in acuity and the body enjoys optimal health.

In *asamprajñāta samādhi,* the three *gunas*—the original principles *sattva, rajas,* and *tamas,* which is to say the principles of cognition, energy, and inertia respectively—have attained perfect balance. This state implies an obliteration of the mind, which cannot continue to exist without the participation of the *gunas.* Three factors cause this balance: *vivekakhyāti* (clear understanding), *parāvairāgya* (the supreme state of detachment), and *nirodha samādhi* (where the sublimated impression of birth is no longer perceived, while the sublimated impression of loneliness prevails). This is *asamprajñāta samādhi.*

Vivekakhyāti is the knowledge that reveals the difference between, on the one hand, an immutable reality that is incomprehensible and radiant (*puruṣa*), and, on the other hand, phenomena in constant change. Ultimate knowledge, produced by *sattva* at its highest point of saturation, combined with total control, leads to the obliteration of the non-self. This is called *parāvairāgya,* fruit of the realization of *puruṣa* and of *rajas* at their highest point of expression. It is then that the mind is subjected to *nirodha* (cessation) by the complete absorption of *vṛittis,* which includes the feeling of self, a stage of *mahat.* It is designated by the term *nirodha samādhi,* which comes from *tamas* in its highest form.

Vivekakhyāti, parāvairāgya, and *nirodha samādhi* are actually three facets of a single state in which the three gunas exert their maximum force before, so to speak, losing their individuality and becoming united in an unmanifested state. This state indicates that the mind has now ceased representing the world to itself and experiencing it as we customarily do, in order to return to its origin, *prakṛiti,* which is a state of balance of the three gunas in which the metempiric being, the supraconsciousness (*puruṣa*) is revealed. At the term of a long spiritual journey, the jīvātman experiences the merging into the ultimate reality in

*Compare with Heraclitus's wisdom, which is pregnant to seekers of Truth: "The hidden harmony is better than the visible" (Fragment 55).

nirvikalpa samādhi, the yogic final realization of Brahman (Parama Śiva) and its three inherent attributes: the power of Being, supreme Consciousness, and supreme Bliss, or *sat cit ānanda.*

The "Royal Way"

The entire process of mental concentration, whatever its stages, applications, methods, and results, has been scientifically dealt with in the discipline of Raja Yoga. It is not possible to reach *asamprajñāta samādhi* other than by the methods that are appropriate for it. It is precisely this form of *samādhi* that is characteristic of Raja Yoga.

Not all Yoga practitioners manage to practice these higher forms; far from it. Only the most advanced adepts can do so. For others, the practice of Haṭha Yoga is a condition sine qua non. It is extremely difficult to reach a mental state where a chosen object of concentration can occupy the mind with clarity, where the very feeling of ego disappears. Nor is it simple to reach a mental state that is favorable to the practice of *dhāraṇā* and *dhyāna,* which are deep levels of concentration. In the majority of cases, experimentation shows that it is very difficult to create a sufficiently deep mental state.

Concentration becomes easier if it is reinforced by suitable physical exercises. Indeed, the mind is made so that it functions using the body, and depends on the state of the body. The dependence of the mind on the body persists up to a very high level of mental concentration. This is why it is important, as long as this level has not been reached, not to neglect the physical. It is in this regard that Haṭha Yoga is so important.

In order to reach a deeper state of concentration, the mind's activity must constantly be improved, which is much more difficult if the mind is "blocked" by an unstable and imperfect body. The lack of balance between the body and the mind can lead to conflicts. Progress in concentration is then seriously inhibited. The refinement of the mind must occur at the same time as that of the body. In that regard, Haṭha Yoga, with its internal cleansing, energizing, normalization of physical and mental functions, and its goal of refining the body and mind, brings us invaluable help. Certain postures, processes of purification, breath control exercises, together with an appropriate diet, to name a few measures, support this discipline.

Mantra Yoga and Laya Yoga

Relatively simple methods have been elaborated in the disciplines of Mantra Yoga and Laya Yoga. In the former, a *mantra,* the potential force of a sound, facilitates the reaching of a higher level of mental concentration. A *mantra* is used in its audible form (*vaikhari*). Using special methods, in particular *japa*—the iteration of an initiation-given *mantra*—the practitioner's ultimate goal is to break the audible sound wall, by which various internal forces are stimulated and from which will emerge two new dimensions, consisting of a super-sound along with the revelation of a higher spiritual consciousness (*devatā*). A beginner first practices the *mantra* in order to learn how to control *dhāraṇā.* It has been determined that the minimum time the mind needs to maintain an image is exactly one seed *mantra* (*bīja mantra*), which, used correctly, presents to consciousness a form of sound that repeats at regular intervals. The shorter these intervals, the more concentration gains depth. The meditator's *mantra* finally becomes an unbroken sound. It is then that the mind enters *dhyāna,* the stage where awareness of *devatā* is reached.

In genuine traditional practices of Yoga, the selection of an appropriate *mantra* (generally consisting of a single or multiple phonemes with no linguistic meaning) is crucial for the practitioner. To be workable, a *mantra* must be duly imparted via *dīkṣā* (initiation) by a genuine guru to a qualified *cela* (student), except for commonly used *mantras* like *aum, śanti,* and so on. *Mantras* that are acquired from books or other sources apart from the guru will not do for the purpose of raising the *mantra's* latent powers. This notion of the guru's indispensable role for success in *japa* practice is a recurring theme in yogic tradition. In modern times, it has been exemplified by Sri Aurobindo, Sri Ramana Maharshi, Sri Ramakrishna, and Sri S. S. Goswami, whose respective gurus were typically modest yogi(ni)s who never received fame commensurate with that later accorded to their *celas.*

In Laya Yoga, a very effective system was developed to reach *dhāraṇā-dhyāna-samādhi*. The method aims at a dissolution of ordinary subject-object consciousness, which leads to an extraordinarily refined and radiant form of consciousness called Kuṇḍalinī. The Kuṇḍalinī is then maintained in certain supraphysical centers (*cakras*) inside the spinal column. This mental process ends in the transition of *dhāraṇā* into *dhyāna* that, in the dissolution of the Kuṇḍalinī, later develops into *samādhi*.*

Postures for Concentration

When we wish to perceive a blurred object or examine something attentively, the body and sight are fixed, immobilized. The very first condition of concentration is the absolute immobility of the body. When it is moving, its vibrations are slower and each one of its parts is less stable. In such a case, the body is hardly suited to mental concentration. Indeed, the instability of the body and the presence of vibrations that are too slow have a negative influence on the mind, which under such conditions cannot become stable. We should add that in order to develop concentration at the levels of *dhāraṇā, dhyāna,* and *samādhi* respectively, it is not enough to keep the body motionless. It should also be placed in a particular concentration posture, the *āsana,* which has multiple advantages.

According to Yoga, the body continues to produce vibrations that oppose mental concentration for as long as the parts of the body intended to produce intense muscular effort are not voluntarily put out of operation. The function of the legs is to produce an intense muscular effort, for example running, during which all the limbs and organs of the body collaborate with the muscles. These activities must be controlled with the assistance of a cross-legged posture. This position makes the body more stable and also contributes to strengthening the will. These two factors facilitate mental concentration.

The arms are also instruments of action, and are specially designed

*A detailed exposition of Laya Yoga is presented in Sri S. S. Goswami's masterwork, *Layayoga* (Inner Traditions, 1999).

for the execution of more complicated movements. They must also be kept motionless during a concentration exercise. For this reason, the pupil adopts the Dhyāna Mudrā posture, in which the right hand is placed on the left hand, palms turned upward, close to the body in front of the abdomen.

Another even more important characteristic of a concentration posture is the maintenance of the trunk in an absolutely vertical position, with the back straight. The rib cage is raised, the abdomen (belly) slightly drawn in, the head straight, and the whole body relaxed. Sitting down with a straight torso is, physiologically, an ideal position for the body. Such a posture is thus beneficial for mental concentration.

It is absolutely necessary that breathing and blood circulation are in no way blocked during the concentration exercise. When the body is motionless, the position of the diaphragm in the thorax, its capacity to pump the air into the lungs, and the tonic contraction of the abdominal muscles play an important role. If the chest subsides, the diaphragm does the same, in the direction of the initial position of inhalation. The margin of movement of the diaphragm is noticeably reduced and, consequently, so is its capacity to pump air into the lungs. The position of the abdominal organs is also modified, thus creating a slight expansion of the abdominal wall. All these negative effects can be avoided if a correct position is chosen and if the muscles are kept in good condition, particularly the abdominal muscles and the muscles allowing dorsal mobility.

For good mental concentration, it is very important to keep relaxed. There are a great number of postures for concentration. In Yoga, three of them are particularly suitable: Sukhāsana (Pleasant Posture), Siddhāsana (Accomplished Posture, posture of the accomplished one), and Padmāsana (Lotus Posture). Mastery of these postures is made possible by regular training. They become usable for concentration when they are mastered with a feeling of comfort.

CONCLUSION

Leading a Modern Life with Classic Yoga

> *True human progress supposes*
> *A harmonious development*
> *Of the body and mind.*
> *In a life without spirituality,*
> *Man wanders with no real goal.*
>
> SRI SHYAM SUNDAR GOSWAMI

The time has gone when the practice of Yoga was considered to be reserved for Hindus and seemed to imply a withdrawal, in India mainly, from a world of survival in which everyone seeks a happiness that continually escapes them. Yoga is a rare phenomenon in the world heritage of cultural expression. It is characterized by an extraordinary vitality and a longevity that challenges human history such as we know it—a tangled fabric of lives tossed about by the ebb and flow of our biosphere: natural disasters, bloody confrontations of civilizations with bellicose intentions, Messianic phenomena founded on successive monarchies, and an unending flood of ideologies. . . . So many elements feed the unfolding centuries during which *Homo sapiens* has struggled unrelentingly in the search for absolute Truth and a happiness that is found at the furthest reaches of human horizons. This struggle, which is as tenacious as our survival instinct, proceeds on the basis of ignorance about our true nature, though we are quite aware of our limitations and the painful certainty of an inescapable end.

However, according to the philosophy of Yoga (*Yogadarśana*), each of us is, by definition, *jīvātman* (*jīva* + *ātman*), that is, of divine nature, with typically human ontological limitations. It is only by a process of transmutation that we are able to become aware of our true nature—without, however, renouncing the various identities that we must assume throughout our journey on Earth: son or daughter, pupil, friend, spouse, father or mother, employer or employee, monk or atheist.

The great adventure of seeking our true identity via the path of Yoga effectively responds to the wise invitation to "Know Yourself." For modern people, it is a sizeable challenge, because it results in having to learn to reconcile our tastes and inclinations and to assume, in a rational manner, our various social obligations, along with the traditional ideal of the yogi, which is none other than an ideal in search of the original Source, expressed in daily life by love and wisdom.

A far cry from dogmatic thought claiming exclusive rights to the Truth, or from salvationist proselytism, Yoga addresses any human being who experiences the need for a grand adventure of introspective research. Its many ways are perfectly suited to the various needs of a candidate. No one is excluded for any reason.

In these times of the globalization of Yoga, one of the major problems that confronts a yogi(ni) candidate is the degree of competence, reliability, and integrity of his or her teacher, whose presence and experience must be carefully considered. The tradition of Yoga teaches that spirituality cannot be an ordinary form of business, with its knowledge put up for sale. It is true that the traditional ashrams of India, together with their pupils and disciples, must ensure a decent level of material comfort for the guru. Nevertheless, the presence and the wisdom of the spiritual guide, the personal experience shared, and the teaching he or she dispenses cannot be the object of any kind of mercantilism.

That this service is inherently free explains the purity, the preservation, and survival of the sacred tradition of Yoga. Conversely, ill-considered commercial exploitation is enough to explain the frequent coming-and-goings of Yoga schools that, like ephemeral comets, emerge and, at once, disappear in the hubbub of new services marketed to an unaware public.

The practice of Yoga is, however, not free. Success requires determination, regularity in practice, and patience regarding the anticipated results. The price to be paid is always determined by the level of ambition of the man or woman who joins the path. Just as in a professional career or even in the commonplace search for happiness, at a higher level sacrifices and trials of all kinds are commonplace.

Leading a modern life with classic Yoga, the author has experienced the very enriching experience of this kind of "Middle Way" or binary life, at the same time "centrifugal" in a dispersed modern society—to which can be added the personal goal to respect family and professional obligations—and in parallel a "centripetal" life of guided, introspective research. A binary life certainly, but its parts never hermetically sealed from one another. On the contrary, it is a true source of richness to be able to establish an osmotic relationship between these two supposedly opposite poles. It was also a chance to receive, in Sweden—the country that adopted me, as it did my master—the qualified teaching of a remarkable man who, although Hindu, was nevertheless conscious of the need for the majority of Westerners to adopt such a "Middle Way," a way that grants as much importance to social life as to the individual's spiritual search.

Without the major changes generated by a regular practice of Yoga under the responsibility of a highly qualified teacher, I would probably never have made a success (self-taught as I was, and in a foreign land) of an international professional career in the world of law (notorious for its conservatism) nor, thereafter, obtained a sought-after post of consultant within the World Intellectual Property Organization (WIPO), one of the specialized organizations of the UN.

Although considered atypical from the outside, my path is on the contrary typical of one searching for the Self, with the usual ingredients of intellectual curiosity set in a climate of rejection, conformity, and modernist philosophy that, once the infatuation with words and arguments has passed, seemed to me speculative verbosity. It is however this dual quest that has brought me both personal development and an exceptional relationship with a sage from another world.

The activities of his school, Goswami Yoga Institute, which was one of the very first in Europe, continued without interuption during approximately three decades in Sweden, solely under the direction of its eponymous founder and, for certain elementary courses, under the responsibility of a close disciple, Mrs. Karin Schalander, who continued to teach until she retired at almost ninety in 2007. When my revered teacher passed away, in October 1978, I was urged (and I accepted) to pursue Sri S. S. Goswami's own classes until my move to southern France, in 1994. Presently, class instruction in Sweden is entrusted to Mrs. Renée Lord. From shortly after his demise in 1978, Sri Shyam Sundar Goswami's teaching has continued with three weekly classes at the school. Seminars are also offered for established students, in the Swedish capital as well as in Europe, the United States, India, and Kurdistan, with the sole ambition of perpetuating a genuine tradition of the spirit of one great master of Yoga.

Note on the Pronunciation of Transliterated Sanskrit Words

The following are the approximate English equivalents.

a	has the sound of a	in all
ā	has the sound of a	in father
ai	has the sound of ai	in aisle
au	has the sound of ou	in loud
b	has the sound of b	in bar
bh	has the sound of bh	in abhor
c	has the sound of ch	in chapter
ch	has the sound of ch	in chop-house
d	has the sound of th	in there
ḍ	has the sound of d	in soda
dh	has the sound of dh	in adhere
ḍh	has the sound of dh	in red-haired
e	has the sound of ey	in prey
g	has the sound of g	in go

gh	has the sound of gh	in log hut
h	has the sound of h	in hot
i	has the sound of i	in it
ī	has the sound of ee	in see
j	has the sound of j	in job
jh	has the sound of dgeh	in hedgehog
k	has the sound of k	in kind
kh	has the sound of kh	in inkhorn
l	has the sound of l	in lady
m	has the sound of m	in mother
ṁ	has the sound of m	in hum
n	has the sound of n	in no
ṇ	has the sound of n	in not
ṅ	has the sound of ng	in king
ñ	has the sound of ny	in canyon
o	has the sound of o	in molest
p	has the sound of p	in pan
ph	has the sound of ph	in philosophy
r	has the sound of r	in ram
ṛi	has the sound of ri	in river
s	has the sound of s	in saint
ś	has the sound of sh	in shun
ṣ	has the sound of sh	in fish
t	has the sound of t	in pasta
ṭ	has the sound of t	in tie
th	has the sound of th	in three
ṭh	has the sound of th	in anthill
u	has the sound of u	in full
ū	has the sound of oo	in moon
v	has the sound of v	in voice
y	has the sound of y	in yet

Glossary

abhimāna Ego projection onto an object

aham Ego

ahamkāra Identification of the Self with the non-self; our ordinary consciousness

ahimsā Nonviolence, universal love

ānanda samādhi Fourth stage of *samādhi* where the sensory organs are disconnected from objects, and where the subject-object relation starts to disappear; happiness

aparigraha Noncovetousness

asamprajñāta samādhi Last stage of *samādhi;* supraconsciousness; a form of *samādhi* in which the consciousness is not formed by any object, not even the awareness of the individual self

āsana Third discipline of the eightfold path (Aṣṭānga) of Yoga; body posture used for mental concentration or physical control and development

asmitā samādhi Third stage of *samādhi* where the yogi is aware of the Self released of the non-self

Aṣṭānga Yoga Yoga doctrine composed primarily of eight subdisciplines: *yama, niyama, āsana, prāṇāyāma, pratyāhāra, dhāraṇā, dhyāna,* and *samādhi*

asteya Refraining from stealing

ātman The Self, whether or not identified with the Absolute (according to various Hindu schools of thought)

Bhakti Yoga Path of devotion; love of the Divine

Bhastrikā Thoracic hyperventilation

bhoga Sensual pleasure

bhūtas Five potential forces that act on the sensory organs to which they present material forms

Bhūta Śuddhi Mental process intended for awakening Kuṇḍalinī

bīja mantra Concentrated form of sound, its "seed"

brahmacarya Chastity; control of sexuality

Brahman The Absolute, the thrice great (*sat cit ānanda*).

cakra Nonmaterial center of force that is perceivable in a certain state of supraconsciousness

cālaṇā A certain type of movement (distinct from the term *cāraṇā*)

cāraṇā Training method for muscular contraction and control that is complementary to the *āsanas*

cela (or sādhak, śiṣya) Student, follower, practitioner of Yoga

citta Field of consciousness in which the sensory world is reflected

darśana School of thought in India; point of view; auspicious internal or external vision of a yogic ideal (yogi, *naga naga, sāddhu . . .*)

deva deha Ideal of the yogi; radiant, divine ideal; outstanding being

devatā Divinity; revealed spiritual supraconsciousness

dhāraṇā Sixth discipline of the eightfold path (Aṣṭānga) of Yoga; first stage of mental concentration in which the current of mental attention toward a given object is intermittent

dhi Mental faculty of concentration

dhyāna Seventh discipline of the eightfold path (Aṣṭānga) of Yoga; second stage of mental concentration with sustained focusing on a given object

Dhyāna Mudrā Characteristic posture of the hands in mental concentration

dīkṣā Important stage for the disciple candidate who connects to a lineage of spiritual masters or gurus; formal yogic initiation

Dvapara Yuga The third of four divisions of time in Hindu cosmology

ekāgratā State of intensive monofocal thought

gunas Three original principles—*tamas, rajas,* and *sattva*—present in any phenomenon of creation; a force can only be understood when it undergoes a change; initially, we are completely unaware of its existence; the unknown form of this force is *tamas*—the potential principle of inertia; the changing form of this force is *rajas*—principle of energy or transformational principle; the perception-comprehension of its existence, as a result of its changing form, is *sattva*—the principle of cognition

Guru In India, the term has the general meaning of teacher or the restricted sense of one who transmits spiritual knowledge and initiation (*dīkṣā*); spiritual teacher

hamsa Mantric unit (unification) (*ham* + *sa*) of breathing; transcription of the first sound of the *ONG* (or *AUM, OM) mantra* on the sensory level

Haṭha Yoga One of the four fundamental paths of the original Yoga (Mahā Yoga)

idā One of the three principal *nāḍīs;* directional subtle force (on the left-hand side)

īśvarapraṇidhāna Mental concentration emanating and associated with love of the Divine

Jālandhara Bandha Chin Lock; voluntary pharyngolaryngeal obstruction

Jala Vasti Colonic Auto-Lavage; self-cleansing of the colon carried out without mechanical assistance

Jñāna Yoga Raja Yoga–related path based on the philosophical distinction of Self and the ego

jīvātman Being incarnated from the divine essence (*jīva* + *ātman*); human being

Kali Yuga The last of four divisions of time in Hindu cosmology

kalpa Long period of time in Hindu cosmology

Kapālabhātī Diaphragmatic hyperventilation

Karma Yoga One of the forms of Raja Yoga, based on action

kevala kumbhaka Spontaneous retention of the breath

Khecarī Mudrā Advanced Breath Suspension

kumba mela Very ancient Hindu pilgrimage that is held in 4-, 12-, and 144-year cycles, in four different locations

kumbhaka Breath retention (apnea)

Kriya Yoga Path of ritualistic Yoga devoted to the Divine, asceticism, and the study of the sacred writings; made popular by the book *Autobiography of a Yogi,* by Paramhamsa Yogananda

Kuṇḍalinī The Grand Spiritual Potential; spiritual consciousness that is potential or dynamic, and is sublime and radiant

Laya Yoga One of the four paths of supreme Yoga (Mahā Yoga) based on the *cakras* (nonmaterial energy centers) and Kuṇḍalinī; the ultimate science of the *cakras*

lingam Ancient Hindu sacred symbol

mahat The separate self

Mahā Yoga Supreme Yoga; the original Yoga, which consists of eight fundamental disciplines (Aṣṭānga); mental superconcentration (see *asamprajñāta samādhi*)

Mahā Yuga Subdivision of the cyclical system of *manvantara*

maithuna Tantric sexual union included in the five "M"s. See *pañca makāra*

Mani Cālana Muscular exercise developing the trunk and the neck

mantra Sound energy that by a special procedure awakens inner forces and spiritual awareness; in Yoga practice it is a single or multiple phoneme with no linguistic meaning

mantra japa Reiteration of a *mantra*

Mantra Yoga One of the four fundamental paths of original Yoga (Mahā Yoga)

Manu Founding father of humanity in a cosmic cycle

manvantara Cyclical passage of time

mauna Practice of silence

mela See *kumba mela*

Meru Cālana Exercise developing the neck muscles

mudrā Exercise of control; hand posture

Mūla Bandha Anal Lock; exercise of voluntary contraction of the anus

nāḍī Immaterial channel; pranic force of kinetic radiation; that which endures motion

nāḍī cakra Energy field; kinetic force acting through the body

Nāḍī Śuddhi Purification procedure for cleaning and energizing the body in the advanced practice of *prāṇāyāma* aiming at facilitating mental concentration

naga naga (or naga baba, naga sāddhu) Elite ascetic in Yoga

Nirmanu Acts of bodily purification

nirodha Suspension; control of mental fluctuations (*vṛittis*)

niyama Second discipline of Patañjali's eightfold path (Aṣṭānga) of Yoga, which consists of five ethical rules: *śauca, santoṣa, tapas, svādhyāya, īśvarapraṇ-idhāna;* observance of these rules

ojas Vital force derived from *prāṇa*

Padmāsana Lotus Posture

pañca makāra (five "M"s) Sacred Tantric practice based on sociocultural prohibitions, which takes a symbolic direction among orthodox Hindus

parāvairāgya Sublime detachment; capacity to exclude the external world from the mind

pingalā One of the three principal *nāḍīs*; directional force (on the right-hand side)

prakṛiti Perfect balance of the three *gunas: tamas, rajas,* and *sattva*

prāṇa Universal, central, bioenergetic force; exhalation

prāṇa vāyu Energy entity that connects the body to the mind

prāṇāyāma Fourth discipline of the eightfold path (Aṣṭānga) of Yoga; yogic method of breath control

pratyāhāra Fifth discipline of the eightfold path (Aṣṭānga) of Yoga; voluntary mental withdrawal from sensory objects; control of the senses

puja Form of Hindu cultural expression; veneration, worship

pūraka Inhalation

puruṣa Metempiric entity; supraconsciousness; form of consciousness beyond duality that cannot be objectified; the Self

rāga-dveṣa Natural alternation of the attraction of pleasure and its opposite

rajas See *gunas*

Raja Yoga The "Royal Way"; one of the four fundamental paths of Mahā Yoga

recaka Exhalation

retas Male seed used in an advanced method of controlling sexual energy

rishi Sage from Hindu antiquity able "to see" all the Vedas

sādhak Synonym for *cela* and *śiṣya*

sādhana See Yoga *sādhana*

Śakti Force, Power; female aspect of the Divine. See Śiva-Śakti.

samādhi Eighth discipline of the eightfold path (Aṣṭānga) of Yoga; end result of mental concentration. See also *asamprajñāta samādhi, samprajñāta samādhi*

samprajñāta samādhi Intense metal concentration in which the yogi has no more awareness of self; consciousness is illuminated only by the object of concentration, and nothing else; called *samprajñāta* because the known is seen in a extrasensory form; includes four subdivisions: *vitarka, vicāra, asmitā,* and *ānanda*

samyama Highest level of Yoga mastery

sanātana dharma Sacred concept of an eternal order in Hindu thought; unites religion and metaphysics

Śaṇkprakṣalana Total self-cleansing of the intestine

santoṣa Satisfaction

Sarasvatī Cālana Process of awakening the Kuṇḍalinī

sat cit ānanda Being-Consciousness-Bliss

Satya Yuga The first of the four divisions of time in Hindu cosmology; era of truth

ṣaṭ karman Six fundamental acts of bodily purification

sattva See *gunas*

satya Veracity

śauca Cleanliness

śiṣya Synonym for *cela* or *sādhak*

Śiva Supreme Consciousness. See Śiva-Śakti

Śiva-Śakti Experience of the Absolute, beyond the mind, where Power (Śakti) is closely related to Supreme Consciousness (Śiva)

śodhana Internal purification of the body

śruti Revealed writings of the Hindu culture in particular the Vedas, Brāhmaṇas, and Upaniṣads

Śuṣka Vasti Colonic Auto-Air Bath; self-cleansing with air carried out without mechanical aid

Siddhāsana Accomplished Posture

siddhis Extraordinary human powers

sūtra Aphoristic statement from sacred Hindu literature

Sukhāsana Pleasant Posture; easy cross-leg posture also known as the "tailor-posture"

suṣumnā The principal of the three pranic forms (*nāḍīs*)

svādhyāya Spiritual study, including *japa mantra*

Svara Yoga Alternative to *prāṇāyāma,* based on an infradiurnal breathing cycle

tamas See *gunas*

tanmātras Miniaturized form of the *bhūtas,* five in number

tapas Asceticism; specific energy process

Treta Yuga The second of four divisions of time in Hindu cosmology

turīya Fourth state of consciousness beyond waking, sleeping, and dreaming

Uḍḍīyāna Bandha Exercise of abdominal retraction

urdhva-retas He whose seminal flow is reversed

vaikhari *Mantra* in its audible form

vairāgya State of nonattachment to earthly goods

Vajrolī, Vajrolī Mudrā Advanced method of sexual control

Vamana Dhautī Gastric Auto-Lavage; self-cleansing of the stomach carried out with water

Vāri Sāra Alimentary Canal Auto-Lavage; self-cleansing of the intestinal tract, carried out without mechanical assistance

Vāsa Dhautī Gastric Cloth-Cleansing; self-cleansing of the esophagus and the stomach by ingesting and withdrawing a long narrow strip of gauze

Vāta Sāra Alimentary Canal Auto-Air Bath; self-cleansing of the intestinal tract with air, carried out without mechanical assistance

vāyu Kinetic force; active manifestation of *prāṇa*

Veda Knowledge; name given to the four books revealed to the rishis in the time known as Vedic, which contain all divine wisdom. They are the *Ṛigveda, Sāmaveda, Yajurveda,* and *Atharvaveda*

vibhūti Superpower; superhuman capacity

vicāra samādhi Second stage of *samādhi* where the yogi perceives a *tanmātra* or "thatness"

vitarka samādhi First stage of *samādhi* where the yogi perceives a *bhūta* or "essential" as a separate element

vivekakhyāti Differentiating knowledge; form of knowledge where Self and non-self appear as two distinct entities

vṛitti Mental fluctuation by which consciousness assumes the shape of an object

yama Control, abstention; first discipline of Patañjali's eightfold path (Aṣṭānga) of Yoga, consisting of five ethical rules: *ahimsā, satya, asteya, brahmacarya, aparigraha*

yogacittavṛittinirodha Traditional definition of Yoga according to Patañjali's second aphorism; state of mind in which all *vṛittis* cease

Yogadarśana Philosophy of Yoga

Yoga sādhana Path; practice of Yoga

Yoni Mudrā An advanced sexual-control practice

yuga An eon in Hindu cosmology

Index